HOW TO ACHIEVE IMMORTALITY

100 Ways to Create Your Own Legacy for Future Generations

By

Lloyd Silverman

This book is a work of non-fiction. Names and places have been changed to protect the privacy of all individuals. The events and situations are true.

First published by AuthorHouse 09/10/04

ISBN: 1-4184-6467-8 (e-book)
ISBN: 1-4184-2921-X (Paperback)
ISBN: 1-4184-2922-8 (Dust Jacket)

Library of Congress Control Number: 2004092120

Printed in the United States of America
Bloomington, Indiana

This book is printed on acid-free paper.

> *"Whence this pleasing hope, this fond desire, this longing after immortality. Eternity Thou pleasing dreadful thought."*
> **William Shakespeare**

INTRODUCTION

Immortality...Eternity...these words conjure up thoughts of awe and question our very essence. Are our lives simply a brief strut on life's mortal stage, a blip on history's screen, then quickly forgotten? Except for the very few, this is unfortunately the fate of most people. In these pages, I hope to change our "fate", our "destiny." I hope to change our perception of immortality. For those who desire to be connected with, or at least be remembered by their families, their community and/or the world's populace, I dedicate this effort.

Mankind has pondered the notion of immortality since the beginning of time. Human beings have found solace and comfort in their religious, spiritual or philosophical beliefs. Recent technological advances in medicine, genetics and cryogenics complicate the very meaning of immortality. In this book, there are *no* discussions of any of these concepts. I only deal with practical ways for you to achieve immortality.

There are basically two incentives for most people to work towards becoming immortal: (1) most people have families or loved ones and desire to be remembered by them now and far into the future and (2) if given the opportunity, many people would aspire to help people in their community and in the world.

In these pages, I present 100 Propositions for you to consider and act upon to achieve your immortality. They vary greatly in the difficultly of accomplishment. The amount of "immortal impact" you will achieve depends how well and how many you can accomplish.

In Part I, I propose 50 Propositions wherein you can be remembered by countless generations of your family. Thus, you can directly influence future generations of your family for centuries ...perhaps forever.

In Part II, I set forth 37 Propositions, in which if you execute any of these Proposition successfully, you will be able to immortalize yourself or someone you choose, living or deceased in your town, city or state. Some of these Propositions will allow you to immortalize your business, civic organization, or even your pet.

In Part III, I present 13 Propositions to challenge you to become a true "immortal". Successful execution will allow you to reach multitudes of people both nationally and internationally.

It must be emphasized; there are no barriers to prevent you or a family member from becoming immortal. It might be easier to begin at an early age, but at any age you can begin. With some Propositions, having children will benefit your quest for immortality. However, if you happen to be single, childless, pet less, mate less, aged or infirmed, this should not inhibit your ability to achieve immortality. Achieving immortality will not depend on having wealth (though having ample funds will help achieve several Propositions) or being a "celebrity" (most fame is fleeting). Again, there are no barriers if you truly want to be immortal. You or someone you choose can have presence on Earth forever. TRY!

ACKNOWLEDGEMENTS

My dream is to give people the means and support to strive to be remembered for endless generations. These are the people who have helped me fulfill that dream.

My wife, Susan Silverman who never wavered in her help, love and encouragement during the writing of this book. There would be no book without her input and steadfast confidence.

My children, Hollis Silverman, Samantha Silverman, Indee Freas and Rachel Tralongo who believed in my dream and will pass this book on to their children...and on...

My editor, Susan Teich, who worked tirelessly and methodically to see that this was a quality book. The exceptional art, layout and production work was her doing. It's excellence speaks for itself.

My family who are part of the Immortal Solutions family...thank you.

Fay and Sid Silverman, Diane and Bill Blocker, Mollie and Jack Steinberg.

And finally, to all the Board members, officers and friends of Immortal Solutions... Thanks for the help and support.

Barry Chitwood, Henry and Zoe Lake, Kelly and Clint Strand, Bonnie Hixson, Paul Yialouris, Peter Ayer, Jean D'Amato, Ed Hoffman, David Irvin, Gary Nobel, and Big Bob.

Lloyd B. Silverman

IMPORTANT NOTES TO KEEP IN MIND

Note 1: Most how-to books explain how to do something. I generally set out how to accomplish many of the Propositions and in the Appendix, offer you the means to directly aid you in your quest. We will remind you to consult the Appendix to obtain these means. Our products include unique legal forms and an instructional C.D. When it comes to legal documents, you are encouraged to contact your attorney or use our legal resources.

Note 2: Most states have passed a law called the Statute of Perpetuities which limits giving gifts beyond three generations. This antiquated Statute will hopefully be dissolved and may impact on only a few Propositions. However, by establishing a family tradition, it will have no real effect on any of them.

Note 3: Contact us on our website Immortalsolutions.com and E-mail us... Immortalsolutions.com or Immortalsol@aol.com. You will get a reply back... guaranteed. We want you to achieve immortality.

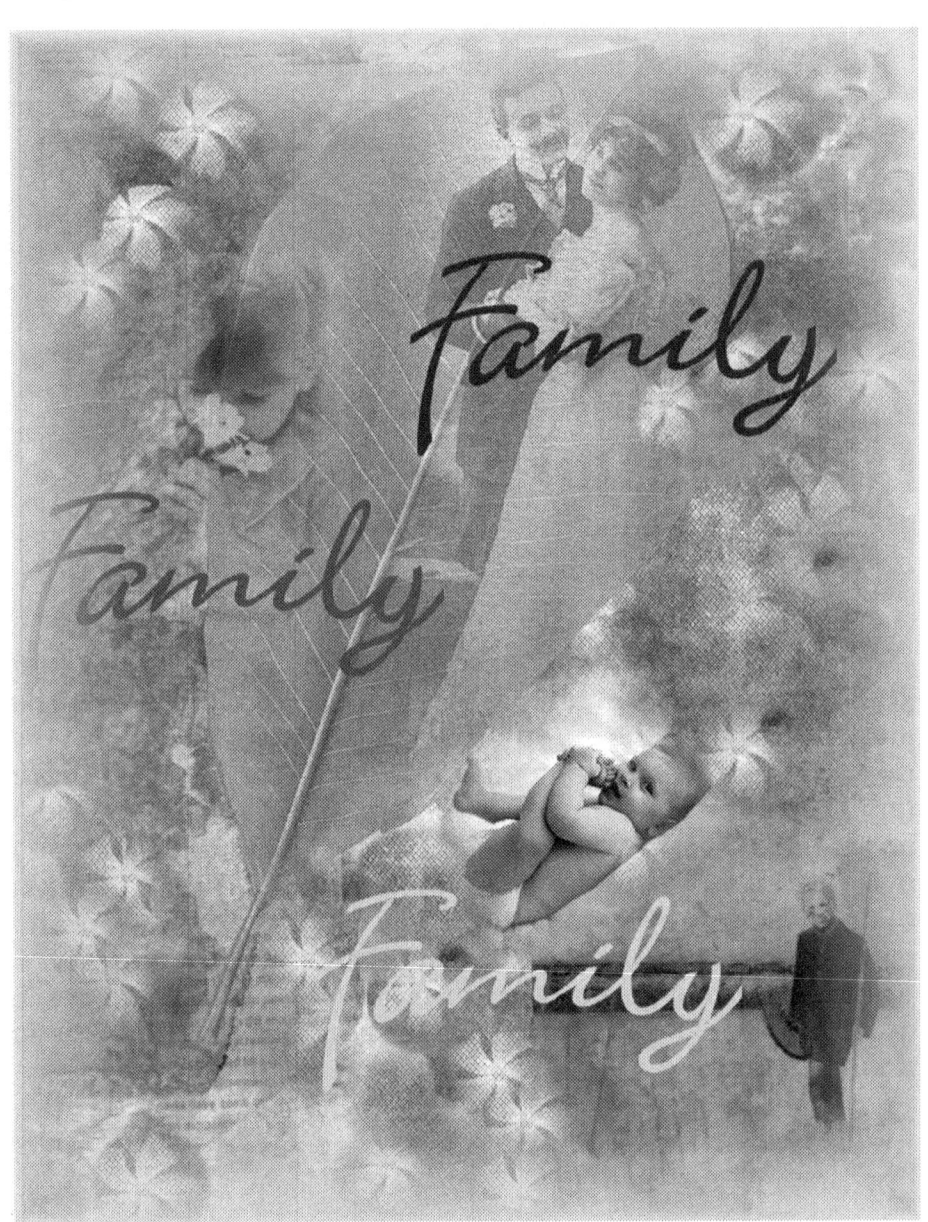

PART I

ACHIEVING IMMORTALITY WITHIN THE FAMILY

In this Part, we have proposed fifty ways, how you or your family can be linked for endless generations. The more Propositions you complete the stronger the possibility you can achieve immortality for yourself, your family, and/or your friends both living and deceased. Most people spend a life time working within the family unit and owe their lives to being part of the family unit. Yet most people have never met or know much of great grand parents who are critical to their existence. Wouldn't you want your great grandchildren or even your great, great, great grandchildren to know about you...They will if you so choose. Begin.

> *"Immortality is the genius to move others, long after you yourself have stopped moving."*
> Frank Rooney, 19th century German Architect

1   CHANGE A NAME

Consider choosing a new first or middle name. Your last name is a legacy in itself. Your name change might incorporate your profession, craft, trade or a hobby. Gardening, golfing or cooking are examples. Choose a name focused on a unique physical trait like red hair. Men who have their father's first name and a Jr. or Roman numeral stamped after their last name, and women, who discard their maiden names after marriage, consider establishing your own tradition.

<u>Examples</u>: Jane Roses Jones, Harry Tees Smith, Dr. Moses Aspirin Lewis, Frank Laws Amigo Esq., Joseph Red McDonald.

- Set out in your will or trust that if future heirs or descendants change their names in your fashion, they will receive a bequest.

True story: In the 1860's, a former Vice Presidential Candidate of the National Vegetarian Party, Carrot Levine, wrote a clause in his will which granted a legacy to males of his bloodline, *if their middle name was the name of a vegetable.* The author knows Carrot's great, great, great nephew. His middle name is <u>Mushroom</u>.

A name change usually requires a simple non-contested court hearing.

2   IMMORTAL WILL

Consider incorporating a family history into your will. File it in Probate Court. The "family history" will is legal. Your property and your history will pass to your descendants for countless generations.

Future generations can use the historical data in your will, even if they receive no legacy. Your history could include: *medical data*, military distinctions, special talents and even family secrets. A photo of yourself can be scanned on to the will. It is legal. Future generations will be fascinated by your physical appearance. Imagine seeing a photo of your great, great, grandparents!

- Your immortal will should be filed in Probate Court; even if it is not used to pass bequests to family members. Filed wills are public documents. Future generations will be able to read your will and learn how your history impacts on their lives. Generally, once a will is filed in court, it will not be destroyed. This document is preserved permanently in court archives.
- If you have an existing will, *add* a codicil, an addition to your will. The codicil can detail your family history. In all states, a codicil can be added to a will. It must be properly witnessed by two people. In some states, you can recite the will on video tape. If you've done so, and you want to add your family history, you will still need two witnesses to make it legal.
- If you have a trust, either a revocable living trust or irrevocable trust, you can include a life history in these documents.

Do you want your will to be read for centuries? Provide a legacy to all family members who read your will. See Appendix to get forms.

> *"Once a new idea springs into existence it cannot be unthought. There is a sense of immortality in a new idea."*
> Edward De Bono 20th century Maltese physician

3 ETHICAL WILLS

Consider writing an ethical will. Unlike the will described in Proposition 2, the purpose of the ethical will is not to pass property. What you can pass, is your wisdom, medical information, family secrets, religious and political beliefs, or anything you want to "say" to your descendants.

An ethical will is appropriate if you have no property to bequeath. You can remember your family, friends and enemies by declaring your love, rendering your apologies, expounding your regrets, and setting your life's record straight by telling someone off. An ethical will can be sent to family and friends before or after death.

- If two people witness your ethical will, file it in Probate Court. There it will be preserved, so that your ancestors can read it.
- If you are giving your heirs property by putting their name on your bank account or as a beneficiary on an insurance policy, then write an ethical will. It will last longer than a monetary legacy.

True story: The origin of ethical wills can be traced to the 19th century Jewish ghettos of Poland. Few residents had assets to pass to their heirs; so ethical wills were given to family members. Original ethical wills can be seen in some large city museums.

With an ethical will, you are giving the ultimate gift...yourself.

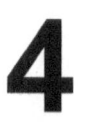

TREASURE HUNT

Consider having "endless" *fun* with heirs, relatives, friends and their descendants. Give them the chance to find the treasure you have hidden. Make your treasure hunt legendary.

Devise clues and riddles. Draw maps and plant evidence. Include treasure hunt hints in your will. Whet the appetite of your heirs and descendants for a competitive adventure. The treasure hunt only ends if someone finds it... perhaps centuries later.

It is essential to appoint reliable executors or trustees and their successors to administer your treasure hunt. They must distribute clues over decades, possibly for centuries. Family member executors might leak clues. A bonded agent could be hired to run your treasure hunt. Remember many buried treasures have never been found.

- Bury or hide your treasure in homes, on private or public land or even under water. Vary the difficultly in finding your treasures. Pack them in hermetically sealed containers. Include in your treasure a photo and letters written to future generations. They certainly will be treasured.
- Use family reunions to announce buried treasure clues.

I (the author) buried a valuable treasure somewhere in the United States. Look on our website for clues. Finder's keepers!

5   LIFE ESTATES

Consider giving your heirs life estates in real property: land, home or condominium. Life estates give heirs, and if you chose their successors, the use of property, but only for their lifetimes. Family members may grumble about your decision: a life estate will prevent them from selling the property. The unpopularity of your choice should not deter you. This *is* a way to establish immortality.

You can use a will, trust or deed to Give a life estate. Set out your logic forcefully; your descendants might continue the tradition of keeping the property in the family. Many states may forbid encumbering real property for more than three of four generations.

- In a life estate, you can restrict *the use of property*. For example, "it may be used *for vacationing only*." You may establish other conditions such as prohibiting your heirs from renting it.
- If an heir breaches your conditions, they could lose their life estate to the next successor.

Keeping property within the family can link generations far into the future. By naming the property... for example, HOUSE OF JONES helps this effort.

6   PASS IT ON

Consider giving your heirs and their successors, a *lifetime use of your most incomparable,* unique personal property. Your ultimate goal here is to pass and preserve your most treasured property for endless generations. Money is *treasured property,* but your heirs could easily squander it in a few years. The property envisioned in this Proposition must be objects large enough or valuable enough, so that they can be preserved and maintained by your trustee and successors. Some examples are an antique car, a rare painting, a gun collection, a rare jewel or a treasured antique.

- Attach conditions on your heir's use of the property. For example, require a rare painting be lent to a museum once a year. Require an antique car to be driven only once a month.

True story: I know a family that passed on a solid gold chess set for six generations. It's amazing no one picked up the pieces and *checked it out.*

Keep your 2000 silver Mercedes sports convertible in the family for centuries.

> *"Man comes and tills the field and lies beneath, and after many a summer dies the swan. Me only cruel immortality consumes: I wither slowly in thine arms, here at the quiet limit of the world."*
> Alfred Lord Tennyson, English 19th century poet

7 RESTRICTIVE COVENANTS

Consider deeding your real property with restrictive covenants attached to the deed. Whether you are selling the property or conveying it to a family member, these covenants or restrictions bind how future owners use the property potentially forever.

For example, if you own a hundred acres of farmland, decide ten acres be used as a baseball field. State this provision on your deed. Instead of growing corn, the game of baseball will be played in the field. Unlike a life estate, your heirs can sell the farmland, but subsequent buyers will need to be careful not to grow corn on home plate.

- This Proposition affects people who own substantial acreage. Restrictive covenants can be placed on residential and commercial property. For maximum impact, name the restricted piece of property for yourself or someone living or deceased. Put that name on the deed.
- Restrictive covenants cannot circumvent zoning laws nor environmental regulations. Due to these restrictions, it is difficult to place restrictive covenants on urban property.
- It is unconstitutional to place restrictions on land, which limits future buyers based on their race, creed, or religion. The United States Supreme Court established this precedent.

Want to establish a hiking trail on your land? Restrict the acreage and name the trail

8

LIFE CHANGING

CONDITIONAL BEQUESTS

Consider inserting life-changing conditional bequests in your will or trust. Your heirs and their successive heirs must fulfill conditions in a specific amount of time. If not, they lose all or part of their legacy.

These conditions should be life altering with significant immortal impact. Appoint reliable trustees/executors and their successors to verify that your specific conditions have been satisfied.

If your heirs refuse or fail to fully accomplish the conditions you've set, they lose their legacy. If that occurs, offer your successor heirs and descendants a chance to succeed. Assert your will from the grave.

- You can attach frivolous conditions to your bequest, such as having your heirs obtain tattoos. This may cause future generations to be similarly tattooed. A condition like requiring your heirs to marry a person of a certain religion or requiring an heir to practice a certain profession is certainly life changing and has far more immortal impact than the tattoo-condition.
- Frivolous or non-frivolous, the immortal goal is to start a tradition, which will last many centuries...perhaps forever.

Have a hankering for your granddaughter to be a surgeon? Not a skull tattoo!

> *"If I should die,' I said to myself, I have left no immortal work behind me, nothing to make my friends proud of my memory, but I have loved the principle of beauty in all things, and if I had time, I would have made myself remembered."*
> John Keats, a 19th century English poet, dead at 26, but forever remembered

9 PRE-NUPTIAL CONTRACT

Consider establishing immortal goals with your intended spouse in an immortal pre-nuptial (before marriage) contract or with your spouse in an ante-nuptial (after marriage) contract. It must be emphasized this is an inspirational document with no legal ramifications, though it can be expanded into a legally binding contract. The ultimate goal of this contract is to sustain your union and to inspire your children, grandchildren and subsequent generations. Be sure to preserve it in a hermetically sealed container!

- You and your mate (*regardless if you marry*) can incorporate your immortal goals in a contract. Hopefully you will refer to it, when continuing your quest to become immortal together.
- In a standard pre-nuptial binding contract, the parties must disclose financial assets and a plan on how to divvy up those assets in case of divorce or death. *The immortal contract here can be incorporated into a standard pre-nuptial contract.* Seek legal advice, if that is your intention.

Like a copy of our inspirational pre-nuptial contract form? See Appendix.

> *"The thought of being nothing after death is a burden insupportable to a virtuous man; we naturally aim at happiness and cannot bear to have it confined to our present being."*
> John Dryden, 17th century English poet

10 WEDDING VOWS

For those contemplating entering into marriage and those already married, who desire to re-recite their wedding vows, consider exchanging *immortal wedding vows*. These vows would be in addition to the traditional wedding vows.

In some classic wedding liturgy, the bride and groom are asked whether they will love and cherish each other "till death do you part". Vow to stay together forever and be remembered by future generations forever. Below are other vows to consider which have an immortal objective. All vows are exchanged under oath.

- Consider the vow to be together for eternity.
- Consider the vow to preserve your life histories for future generations.
- Consider reciting your vows on each wedding anniversary. Copy them and send them to family members.
- Consider doing all the above, to establish a lasting family tradition.

Preserve a copy of your vows in a burial spear for your descendants to read.

> *"For though they be punished in the sight of men, yet is their hope, full of immortality."* **Solomon, a B.C. King**

11 IMMORTALITY AGENT

Consider contracting with a professional agency or an individual to assist you (and your family) in fulfilling your immortal goals. Your immortality agent can be an established law firm, C.P.A. firm, a lobbyist or a literary or entertainment agency.

When contracting with such an agent, be specific as to your immortal goals. Broad goals are hard for an agent to fulfill. For example, if you want a bridge named after you in your hometown, so state it in the contract. If you're not specific, your agent might secure naming rights for you on an ice bridge in Greenland.

- The agent must be bonded to insure performance.
- It is preferable to contract with an agent while you're alive. However, in your will, you can order your executor/trustee to contract with an immortality agent for yourself or someone living or deceased. Provide for successor agents in case the first agent fails in providing the legacy you have willed.
- An agent should produce many immortal opportunities for you and your family for countless generations. Many families have long relationships with a variety of professional firms and companies. Begin a family tradition retaining a family immortality agent.

You may need an agent to contract with an immortality agent. See Appendix for help.

> *"Perhaps even more important than the curing of specific physical and emotional symptoms is the knowledge that we do not die when our bodies do. We are immortal. We do survive physical death."* **Dr. Brian Weiss, 20th century physician and author**

12 A CINEMATIC HISTORY

Consider producing an oral or autobiographical film. It is preferable that this project be done while you are alive, but if you want your film to be produced or finished posthumously, then give your trustee or executor guidelines as to film length, content, and production quality. Also earmark funds specifically for the project.

In this Proposition, you can star, produce and direct your piece of cinematic immortality.

- Require heirs and descendants to view the film, video, or DVD as a condition to receiving their legacy. Or in other words—bribe them into watching it.
- If you or anyone in the family, living or deceased, have been in a television production, motion picture, taped theatrical production, recital or recorded radio show, make certain a copy or copies are obtained and preserved. In your will or trust offer copies of these tapes and recordings to heirs and descendants. Many generations will want to see them.
- Tape and preserve the birth of your children, baby's first steps, first words, school productions, or religious celebrations and … well, you know what is truly immortal.

Think of future generations…make your own family epic.

> *"If your contribution has been vital, there will always be somebody to pick up where you left off, and that will be your claim to immortality."* Walter Gropius, 20th century German architect

13 IN YOUR OWN WORDS

Consider writing and self-publishing an autobiography and/or a biography of a family member(s) or friend. If necessary, collaborate with a professional writer to improve the manuscript. For immortal purposes, it is essential to include medical and family history. Tawdry family secrets can add a bit of spice. Publish numerous copies of your book for future generations to read.

If you don't have time to write a book, then keep a personal journal. Use archival paper and ink. It will be read and appreciated, forever.

- Provide a legacy in your will or trust for those heirs and descendants who read your book. Your trustee must have proof that they did. Be sure to send your book to the National Library of Congress. They'll keep it forever. Get an ISBN number and copyright it. Contact the U.S. Copyright Office, Washington D.C. for details.
- If you want an autobiography or biography written posthumously, set aside funds in your will or trust. Specify what photos and acknowledgements should be included.

Preserve your book and sign the cover. Only a copy of a preserved published book is Immortal. See Appendix for help in completing this Proposition.

> *"It is immortality, and that alone, which amid life's pains, abasements, the soul can comfort, elevate and fill."*
> Charles Young, 19th century English poet.

14   SAY, "Cheese"

Consider having a bust, oil portrait, or commercial photograph created of you or of another person living or deceased. Marble and bronze busts will last for countless centuries. If properly framed and maintained, oil and water color paintings can exist for innumerable centuries.

Limited funds? Then sit for a professional photograph. A blue ribbon quality, beautifully framed photograph will potentially last forever.

Do not be concerned about being perceived as egotistical. A little ego is essential to attain the stature of being an immortal.

- In your will or trust, require heir(s) and their successor(s) to prominently display your image. No attics or garages, please!
- Many art students are capable of producing fine portraits.
- Contact art schools to commission a portrait from a student artist. Refrain from charcoal or chalk drawings, since they may not retain their quality over many centuries. Heirs and descendants will want to see an accurate picture of your appearance. Say "no" to impressionistic portraits.

Your portrait can last forever. Is that why Mona Lisa is smiling?

> *"Our hope for immortality does not come from any religions, but nearly all religions come from that hope."*
> Robert Ingersoll, American, 19th century orator, philosopher

15 YOU'VE GOT MAIL!

Consider setting up a fund in a will or trust to provide birthday, holiday, and anniversary gifts (money or stock is best) to family members or friends, *after your death*.

Provide personal greetings in your own handwriting. These short messages can be delivered on a schedule set up in your will or trust. You also can send a gift or card on behalf of someone who is deceased. The gifts and cards can be delivered for endless generations.

- **Make trustees/executors and their successors responsible for updating addresses and delivering gifts.**
- **List those bloodlines to be remembered in the future.**
- **Even if your trust becomes depleted, the family tradition will be established. Future generations will hopefully continue what you started.**

True story: A client of mine received a gold pocket watch from his Uncle Bill, for his thirteenth birthday (bar mitzvah). A note read:

"Something to remember me by, Uncle Bill." He knew he had a reclusive uncle Bill, but never met him. The watch was Bill's sole legacy. My client received the watch when he was thirty six. It was lost in the mail. The watch doesn't keep time but he wears it everyday.

Make them remember you...forever.

> *"Reputation, reputation, reputation. O! I have lost my reputation. I have lost the immortal part of myself and what remains is bestial."* **William Shakespeare, 16th century poet and dramatist**

16 | HISTORICAL C.D. OR COMPUTER CHIP

Consider creating a computer disk narrating either your family history, your autobiography or a biography of a family member or friend, living or deceased.

On the disk you can include graphics, data, and philosophy. Reminisces are always interesting. Include any clues to a treasure you buried. Establish a fund so the disk can be updated, preserved, perpetually copied, and distributed to future generations.

With advances in technology, a computer disk or computer chip could last forever. Your voice may be heard forever.

- Your historical computer disk or chip should be preserved in a memorial time canister. [Please see Proposition 28].
- In a will or trust, make a bequest to any family member who annually listens to the disk ...after proving it to your executor or trustee.

True story: Most of us have heard phone-answering messages from people who've passed away....its eerily wonderful. I have several from deceased clients. These kinds of tapes should be preserved.

Load up the P.C. and be remembered far into the A.D.

> *"The nearer I approach the end, the plainer I hear around me the immortal symphonies of the worlds which invite me. It is marvelous, yet simple."* Victor Hugo, 19th century French author

17 ETERNAL WEBSITE

Consider providing in your will or trust, funds to create and update a personal/ family website. The website can feature personal and family photos, oral histories, progress on finding buried treasure and endless stories.

As time passes, the site must be updated with family information to include: births, deaths, marriages and family reunions. Conceivably, your perpetual immortal website will keep future generations "connected" to you forever.

- To achieve the best results, appoint and pay an institutional trustee or executor and their successors, to oversee the project.
- In your will or trust, earmark a fund to provide legacies to those family members who contribute to the website.
- We can only guess what the internet will be like hundreds of years from now. Be sure your website is still included.

Stay forever connected! See our immortal website: ImmortalSolutions.com

18 PRESERVE YOUR PAPER

Consider laminating or hermetically sealing your papers and documents for future generations. Preserve newspaper clippings, school documents, letters, educational degrees, military papers, medical records, children's letters, holiday cards, poems, photos, drawings, recipes and public records...your historical paper.

Create a paper history. The documents should be preserved in non-rusting, fireproof, metal containers or thick plastic albums which should be placed in a large memorial canister.

- Monetary incentives should be included in your will or trust to induce heirs and descendants to preserve, update and show their scrapbooks to future generations.
- On paper, paste some of your baby's hair, child's teeth or other DNA substances and enshrine it in a scrapbook.

True story: My client lived overseas. His parents died and he phoned a moving company to remove and safeguard the contents of his deceased parents' house and discard the garbage. The mover tossed out the papers and photos. My clients lamented, "The mover stored the garbage and tossed away my life."

Turn your history and family history into art, by making your scrapbook art.

19 WHOSE PROPERTY IS IT, ANYWAY?

Consider preparing a list of personal property to give to relatives and friends, and attach it to your will or a trust. In most wills, the deceased will instruct their executor (often the children) to distribute their personal property *in their discretion*. They assume the children will complete this task without quibbling. This decision is frequently imprudent and can result in an immortal family feud.

It is recommended you send some remember-me type items, to friends and relatives, while you are alive. Inscribe your name on the inside of book covers and engrave it on metal objects. As long as the object lasts, your name lasts.

- Have your trustee/executor send letters to beneficiaries, urging them to keep the items they received and pass them on to the next generation. In your will/trust motivate them monetarily. Urge each generation to follow this tradition.
- There are scores of lawsuits, involving siblings fighting over personal property. So make a list!

True Story: There is a Florida case where two sisters spent twenty thousand dollars fighting over the possession of a painting worth a hundred dollars.

Your distant relatives may not know who you are. Let them find out!

21

> *"Without a belief in personal immortality, religion is like an arch resting on one pillar or like a bridge ending in an abyss."*
> Max Muller, 19th century German philosopher

20 TIMELESS MEMORIAL

Consider creating a permanent memorial to honor yourself or anyone alive or deceased. Honor your children, spouse, parents, grandparents, pets or friends. It's important the memorial be lasting. Temporary memorials, like roadside memorials, vanish quickly.

Memorials can be statues of yourself or any person or a sculpture of an object that is dedicated to yourself or anyone. In your will or trust, provide monetary gifts to entice future generations of family and friends to visit the memorial.

- Timeless memorials can vary in size. Place objects linked with each person in the memorial itself or under it. From baby hair to a death certificate....provide as many objects as possible.
- Use materials that will last forever. Treated rock, tungsten, marble, or bronze are such materials. Heavy plastic and certain treated wood can be used. Use the best for the people dearest to you!
- Plant memorials on your homestead or on the honoree's property. Perhaps, purchase land for all memorials or plant them on remote public lands, underwater venues or caves.

Note the location of your memorials in your will or trust.

There are statues in existence from biblical times...yours could last that long.

> *"Was this the face that launc'd a thousand ships, And burn the topless towers of Illium? Sweet Helen, make me immortal with a kiss!*
> Christopher Marlowe, 16th century English poet, dramatist

21 | RELIGIOUS SHRINE

Consider building a religious shrine to honor your family, yourself or anyone, living or deceased. The religious shrine envisioned might range in size from a small hut to a structure large enough to accommodate a congregation. Regardless, the shrine should be built with the strongest affordable materials. The objective is to construct a shrine that will last forever. Marble, granite and treated rocks are materials that should be considered.

If you desire to build your shrine as an addition to an existing church or temple, be sure the religious institution will guarantee your immortal goals. Building a shrine, modest or grand, will insure your control and your immortality.

- In your will and/or trust, instruct the trustee/executor and their successors to arrange for a prayer, poem or statement to be recited on the anniversary date of your death or the death of someone you designate. A holiday or birthday would also be appropriate dates. The exact location of your shrine should be noted in these documents.
- In your shrine, store photographs, DNA samples of yourself and your family, personal items, and any religious items.

Build a religious shrine that your ancestors will visit for centuries.

22 GATHER TOGETHER

If you reside in a condominium, a rental, housing project, retirement home, nursing home, trailer or co-op, consider lobbying your Board of Directors, landlord or developer to set aside land to plant small permanent memorials honoring deceased loved ones and/or yourself.

The concept of immortalizing might be a powerful inducement for developers and landlords to attract people to buy or rent their property. Small memorials or religious artifacts will give comfort to the bereaved and the resident, *if the hallowed property is permanently maintained*. It will also give to each person so honored, an indelible mark of immortality.

- In the lobbying effort, induce landlords, condo boards or developers to allow memorials for pets.
- Note the location of your memorial in your will or trust. This information is essential, so heirs and descendants will be able to visit. Be sure to store at least a photograph, DNA sample and a letter inside the memorial or shrine.
- If you are the leader of this lobbying effort, your effort might be copied by other groups giving you a special immortal laurel.

Help many band together, so that many can be remembered... forever.

> *"With our lives we give life. Something of us can never die, we move in the eternal cycle of darkness and death, of light and life."*
> The New Union Hebrew Prayer Book

23 AN IMMORTAL COLLABORATION

Consider organizing your family and/or friends. Collaborate on executing an immortality project, giving all who do participate... immortality. Choose one or many of the immortal missions noted in this book. A simple scrapbook, a charitable enterprise or a multi-family film are immortal projects your group could plan and execute successfully.

In addition to a family joint effort, seek out members of a church, temple, civic, business or support group, to form your collaborative immortality venture. Those who participate will be spiritually uplifted.

- In each participant's will or trust, set out details how the project(s) will be continued and maintained. Bequests should be coordinated and given to future heirs and descendants who continue the work. This is critical for the project(s) to be perpetuated forever.
- Families can be linked for centuries, by maintaining immortal projects. This effort could possibly promote marriages among the families and for certain, century old friendships.

A forever group bonding tradition. Sounds wickedly cozy.

24 HALLOW THE HALLS

Consider lobbying your local religious institution to initiate innovative ways to promote and sustain parishioner immortality. In most religious institutions, name-only plaques hang dispassionately on the walls. Often names are etched on windows, doors and inside prayer books. Parishioners will gain only a modicum of immortal impact, spending money on these ineffectual tributes.

Persuade religious leaders to create a sacred area to honor the deceased. In the area, provide an opportunity for families to permanently house interactive family time capsules. Parishioners can place small items like hair or a photo of a deceased family member into the capsules. Future generations can add items and periodically view them.

- Lead the movement. Have your religious institution establish a remembrance room, garden or building dedicated to honor the deceased. Set a serene and respectful atmosphere for visitation.
- Besides time capsules, lobby to have a variety of biographical plaques and photos placed in this hall of remembrance. Stay away from bland plaques that are virtually ignored.

Halls of Remembrance can bond families with their religious institution forever.

> *"They eat, they drink and in communion sweet. Quaff immortality and joy."* **John Milton 17th century English poet**

25   BE CLONED

Once viewed as science fiction, cloning is becoming a reality in our time. So, consider being cloned. If one believes in the miraculous possibility of a second life, have a clause inserted in your will to affirm this desire.

Take steps to preserve your DNA. Hair or teeth are genetic material you can store for future use. You also can store your blood and human tissue within a private storage facility.

Perhaps, in the future, only those who have executed a clear desire to be cloned in their will or trust, will be rewarded with an opportunity for a "second life". Likewise, only those who clearly rebuke the idea, in writing, will deter relatives from actually cloning you. Want to be frozen, just to be revived in the future? These are all possibilities!

- If you choose to be cloned, leave enough funds in a trust for that purpose. Do not expect your ancestors to spend money to clone you...it may be expensive.
- See Appendix to find information on tiny time capsules that can be worn and keep one's DNA far into the future.

I do not endorse nor censure human cloning or being frozen and revived. These are now "long shots" at a second life, but in the future...?

> *"Not all the subtleties of metaphysics can make me doubt a moment of the immortality of the soul, and a beneficent providence. I feel it, I believe it, I desire it, I hope it and will defend it to my last breath."*
> **Jean Rousseau, 18th century Swiss philosopher**

26 INSURANCE CHALLENGE

Consider purchasing life insurance or a planned annuity policy, that will challenge your beneficiaries to complete a legendary feat or project. If they succed, they will receive the insurance proceeds after your demise. If they fail ...nothing.

The insurance company will determine if the challenge has been met. Insurance companies are dispassionate. They concern themselves with only the facts. Policy benefits will be a major motivation for a beneficiary to meet the test. Note: It may be difficult to find an insurance company willing to write such a policy. They may be afraid of lawsuits, since they will be judging your descendants' performance and a negative determination might make your descedants angry.

- Make your challenge extremely difficult to complete but not impossible. You don't want the insurance company to hold the benefits for centuries...or do you?

Want your artifacts buried on Mt. Everest or the North Pole? They'll do it or lose it!

27 IMMORTAL BUSINESS

Consider naming your business with your name or the name of someone living or deceased. Pass the business to family members or employees on the condition the business name never changes.

Business names like Hershey, Ford, Edison, Fox, or Warner are just a few immortal names. Many names become part of a city or town and are immortalized in the names of streets and civic institutions. A family's name attached to a business has the potential of maximum immortal impact.

- Pass a corporate resolution that the business or firm's name must always remain even if sold. Future buyers must be made aware of the resolution and must agree to abide by it in the contract for sale.
- Specify in your will or trust that heirs and their successors will only inherit the business, if the name remains.
- Many professional firms (law, accounting etc.) keep the founders names as the firm's name. If you work for such a firm, consider starting your own firm and make it immortal.

True story: Like black olives? Check out Black Pearls. On the label, is the story of the Munro family complete with a picture of the grandfather. This is an example of how family names become immortalized. To be clear, I don't know anyone from the Munro family, but their black pearls are quite tasty.

What name do you think has more immortal impact, McDonald or Burger King?

> *"Nothing short of an eternity could enable man to imagine, think and feel and to express all they have imaged thought and felt. Immortality which is the spiritual desire, is the intellectual necessity."*
> **Edward Bulwer-Lytton, 19th century English novelist**

28 | A MEMORIAL TIME CANISTER

Consider burying or preserving a "part" of yourself and/or your family into a memorial canister. Canisters can range in size, from small safes to large vaults. The canister should be made from alloys impervious to time such as: titanium, anodized aluminum with nickel platting, or marble.

Place items in your canister: photographs, mint money, medical records, videos, family heirlooms and letters on archival paper. Include a part of yourself and family members, DNA items such as hair or teeth. This receptacle must be hermetically sealed. If you build your canister, prepare the container so its contents will last indefinitely. See Appendix for help.

- In your will/ trust, note the location of the canister. A buried canister is worthless if it cannot be found. Be sure you give trustworthy family the keys to the vault.
- If you own a business or head a non-profit corporation, bury a canister and immortalize your business.

A few companies sell canisters. They are expensive. See Appendix for our alternative.

> *"Those who hope for no other life, are dead even for this one."*
> Johann Goethe, 19th century German philosopher

29 HAMMER A SPEAR

Consider hammering or burying a memorial spear (time capsule) into your or your family's "historical places".

Memorial spears are substantially smaller than the canister, but must be large enough to hold these items: a photo, a message for the future, a DNA sample (hair) and a small treasure such as a coin.

Construct (or buy) a spear so it is pointed on one side and flat on the other. With this design, it is easier to place into cliff crevices, tree stumps, stone fences or into hard ground.

- A smaller version of the spear may be planted beside or into the grave, placed in a grave or mausoleum vase or inserted into some gravestones. It can contain a prayer, poem and DNA. In this way, the living can be linked with the deceased forever. In your will, mention the location of the small spear. If it has been removed or moved, the grave may have been tampered with.
- If spears are nickel platted and water tight, place them in the ocean or a lake etc. Instead of scattering human or pet ashes into the wind, bury them in a spear.

See Appendix to find out information about the time capsules described here.

30 SPIRITUAL MEDIUMS AND PAST LIVES

If you believe in spiritual mediums or spiritual advisers, then consider setting aside money in your will or trust to arrange for future spiritual contact. Set out specific instructions on how contact is to be made and with whom.

A spiritual challenge should tantalize future generations to continue the tradition of medium intervention. Perhaps, family reunions will occur in another dimension.

- Your executor or trustee and their successors should be given names of mediums to use for the "crossing over" process.
- If you believe in reincarnation or a spirit filled world, be sure to leave some personal property or DNA in a burial spear. It may aid the "medium" in making contact with you in the future.
- If you have experienced a near death experience, an out of body journey, life regression therapy, time travel, or have had contact with a variety of apparitions like shadow people and ghosts, detail these experiences in your will, trust or auto- biography. Challenge future descendants to do the same. (See Proposition 39).

Look in the Appendix for" the oculus"...it may help you connect.

31 | A LEGENDARY BURIAL

Consider drawing up a death plan. If you want your last ride on the mortal merry-go-round to be legendary, then so instruct your executor in your will. Be sure to specify your final resting spot. This idea may seem depressing, but by setting out your wishes, your heirs cannot bicker over your arrangements. Your choice could create a strong family custom followed by an infinite number of generations

Death plans must be detailed. Lay it out as if you'll be attending your own funeral. Write your own eulogy. Name the person who will deliver it.

- Some exotic final send off might be: bagpipes at dusk, a Viking send-off via a burning raft, an anything-goes wake, or a grave site service where memorial stones are left in tribute.
- If cremation is your choice, specify how your ashes are to be preserved or scattered. Instruct your executor/ trustee to save some ashes for a burial spear and remembrance stones.
- If you're not confident that a family member will execute your death plan correctly, contract with an agent.

True story: My client kept his burial plans secret. His religious belief mandated that he be buried. He passed away without a funeral. His two children were not notified. They have searched to find his remains for a decade. No luck.

See Appendix to learn about remembrance stones that can be used in a burial service.

32 CLONE A PET

Consider cloning your beloved pet. Store your pet's DNA material in a burial spear or canister. This will enable your descendants to have your pet's DNA, so that it can be cloned in the future. Cloning your animal can link you to countless generations.

Your terrier could be the same one owned by your great, great, great, great, great, great grandson or granddaughter. An immortal legacy!

- Place a clause in your will, exhorting family members, heirs and descendants to clone their animals. If they do, they'll receive a legacy. Someday soon, cloning will be a reality, so prepare for it. If you are against cloning, consider giving a legacy to those in the family that keep the same breed of animal or an animal that closely resembles your pet.
- Take a quality photograph or have a portrait done of your pet. Hopefully, future generations of your family will preserve it and do likewise with their pets.
- Instill in future generations, the desire to continue the tradition of having a specific pet as part of the family. Consider consulting with a taxidermist.

Pets have short lives...consider extending those lives, hundreds of years.

> *"Because I could not stop for Death, He kindly stopped for me. The carriage held but just ourselves, And immortality."*
> Emily Dickinson, 19th century American poet

33 IT'S not just ASH...

If cremation is your "final choice," or the choice of family, then consider "recycling" the ashes instead of scattering them in the wind. You and loved ones can be remembered and have presence on earth forever, if ashes are kept and preserved.

Don't store ashes in an urn or coffee can (which likely will get lost when moving.) In your will or trust arrange for your ashes to be used. Arrange to have an artist mix your ashes or the ashes of a loved one, with paint and order the paint used in a portrait. Ashes can be mixed with clay, and a statue can be created. Ashes can be mixed with hot metal and cast into a sculpture. At the very least, store ashes in a canister or spear. Bury the spear in a special place away from others, have your name or a loved one's name engraved on it.

- Provide a legacy to all descendants who preserve their ash portrait or statue. Encourage heirs to follow your lead... tradition!
- While alive, cut your hair and nails, burn them and store the ash or integrate them into art projects.
- Your ashes or a loved one's can be put into a stone or other jewelry. It should be worn over the heart. In many cultures wearing a beloved's ashes brings good luck.

"Ashes to ashes"...forever and forever. Please see Appendix for our help.

> *"There is only one way to get ready for immortality and that is to love this life and live it as bravely and faithfully and cheerfully as we can.*
> Henry Vandyke 19th -20thcentury U.S. poet and educator

34 INSPIRED GRAVESTONE

Consider creating and designing a unique gravestone or burial chamber. If it's startlingly distinctive, descendants will visit it for centuries.

To motivate your descendants, drill your stone with a special chamber which should contain: DNA (hair), photographs, a message to the future, a clue to a buried treasure and a CD or computer chip with family and medical history. The stone chamber should be sealed or locked. Items must be retrievable, so they can be viewed or borrowed.

In addition, commission a likeness of yourself or engrave an immortal epitaph on the stone. If one prefers a mausoleum, financially motivate your family to place remembrance stones into the mausoleum vase.

- Be sure to note the location of your gravestone and other family gravestones in a will or trust.
- Replace or augment old stones of relatives or friends.
- As an alternative to drilling, affix a permanent locked holder to the outside of the stone or mausoleum to store a photo, DNA material or letter. However, a drilled stone is less likely to be tampered with, easier to maintain and can hold more.

Shop for a cemetery that will allow gravestone augmentation. It won't be easy.

> *"Some for renown, on scraps of learning dote,*
> *And think they grow immortal as they quote."*
> Edward Young, 18th century English poet

35 TOGETHER FOREVER

Consider constructing a family memorial park (cemetery). If possible, move interred relatives from other places. Why be buried forever with strangers?

In an urban area, land costs and zoning restrictions will make a family cemetery an expensive venture. Some cemeteries have expensive family plot areas. A rural setting will be far less costly and it is likely there will be few, if any, government restrictions.

- Public, private and religious affiliated cemetery owners and administrators make the rules governing burial on their land. By establishing a family cemetery, your family and their descendants make the rules. (See Proposition 34).
- Establish a fund in your will or trust for perpetual security and maintenance.
- Consider building a memorial to your ancestors who are not interred anywhere, those lost in war or in the Holocaust.
- Throughout the ages, there have been abundant reports of spiritual sightings. You should not discount the possibility of a spiritual world. It is possible!

True story: Early in my legal career, I visited many small farms in Kansas and Missouri. Many farms had family cemeteries. Several farmers reported seeing spiritual activity at a variety of burial sites.

A family together, today and always…

> *"Physical immortality is within sight. There are people living today who may extend their life spans indefinitely"*
> **Dr. Ben Bova, 20th century American scientist**

36   PERPETUAL VISITS

In your will or trust, consider enticing your heirs, friends and descendants with monetary rewards, if they visit your grave, family cemetery or any immortal memorial you designate. To ensure that the visit might become a family tradition, schedule it on a religious or a secular holiday, on a significant family anniversary or birthday.

Request your descendants to leave a *remembrance stone* or small time capsule with a certain prayer or message in it. Unlike flowers, a stone lasts forever. See information on *remembrance stones* in the Appendix.

- Instruct your trustee/executor and their successors on how to verify the visit was made. No visit, no reward. (Reread Proposition. 11)
- If a religious service is to be held at the time of the visit, donate a perpetual legacy to a religious institution. The bequest should be conditioned upon a member of the clergy conducting the service.
- If a tradition of generational visiting can be established without a bounty, that would be special! How you conducted your life may influence how many people will visit you.

Establish a lasting family tradition of generations visiting generations, even if it has to be induced with monetary gifts.

> *"A letter always seemed to me like immortality because it is the mind alone, Without corporeal friend."*
> Emily Dickinson, 19th century American poet

37   WRITE A LETTER

Consider writing letters...lots of them. Instruct your trustee or executor and their successors to mail them "periodically" *after your death*. Do it annually, once in a decade, or perhaps every quarter century! Have the letters mailed to heirs, friends, descendants, distant relations, business associates and civic institutions. Send letters to lost loves and present day enemies. Send letters filled with predictions and individual hopes. Perhaps, send one to your local newspaper. That would be a memorable "letter to the editor."

You should contract with a bonded firm, to mail the letters and update the addresses upon your demise. The bond will insure their continued performance.

- Letters can be installments of your life history.
- Establish a tradition of family letter writing, which will continue forever.
- Leave letters in your memorial canister or spear. Use acid resistant paper, archival inks and a wax seal. These precautions will help preserve the letters for centuries.

Write a letter to one's great, great, great, great, great grand daughter... Now!

> *"The joys of marriage are the heaven and earth, Life's paradise, the soul's quiet, sinews of concord, earthly immortality, eternity of pleasures..."* John Ford, 17th century English writer

38   FAMILY REUNIONS

Consider setting aside funds in your will/trust to promote and persuade family members to participate in reunions now and in the future.

Family reunions can be scheduled on the date commemorating a religious or secular holiday, a significant date in the family's history, the date of a family member's death or of your own passing.

In your will/trust the definition of *family* must be clearly defined. Should in-laws be allowed? By perpetuating family get-togethers, hopefully they will keep the family united forever.

- In your will/trust, set out family reunion details such as: location, how often it should occur, what expenses the estate or trust will pay and if a traditional prayer should be recited.
- To insure reunion attendance, offer a monetary incentive to attendees. For some families, it will be necessary.
- Not interested in *family reunions*? How about a perpetual reunion of your civic, religious, or social club members? The same financial incentives for attendance should apply, as well as, a tribute to the facilitator...you.

True Story: A family reunion I attended as a guest was always held at the Ohio State and Michigan football game. Go Buckeyes! Go Wolverines!

Set up a perpetual bash. Prepare a tailgate party. Sounds like fun!

39   SPIRITUAL VISIT

Do you believe in spiritualism? Consider placing a clause in your will or trust announcing when and where you will "reappear." If you decide to reappear at a family soiree, give monetary incentives to those who attend. Set aside money in a trust or will to cater the affair. The event could be eerily exciting.

There have been multitudes of "spiritual sightings" throughout the ages. Why not yours? And even if you don't happen to appear that year...try ...try again...forever.

- Does appearing in a dream count?
- Who qualifies for a spiritual legacy? You decide!
- Please see Proposition 30.

True story: When I headed a legal aid program in the Bronx, New York, my no-nonsense, extremely honest secretary mentioned she once was visited by an Indian spirit in the South Bronx. Though the spirit didn't say anything and she knew no Native Americans, she became an activist for Native American rights. She also told me her mother often saw ghosts walking the South Bronx streets late at night. That I believe!

There are a plethora of reports and books on people having "contact' with a spirit. So....Boo!

> *"Death is a very dull, dreary affair, and my advice to you is to have nothing whatever to do with it."*
> W. Somerset Maugham, 20th century British novelist quoted in his book, <u>Why Die? A Beginner's Guide to Living Forever</u>

40 BUILD A MT. RUSHMORE

Consider building a single monument to honor yourself, a loved one (alive or deceased) or to your family. Build it big, unusual and solid. Use materials like treated wood (black walnut is excellent), bronze or marble, which lasts forever.

In this Proposition, monuments do not include mausoleums, crypts, cemetery markers, religious shrines or the smaller timeless memorials (see Proposition 20). If you desire your memorial to be built after death, set out specific details in your will/trust. Be sure to allocate a sufficient bequest to build your dream memorial.

- Examples of monuments you might consider: a mini Mount Rushmore with your face or faces of your family, a large fresco or mural with images of yourself or family, or an unusual home or historic building crammed with your furnishings…include a portrait. Be sure to name the building and place a <u>restrictive covenant</u> in the deed so the name is preserved. Perhaps, the home will receive the designation as an historic home and be maintained by the State. (See Propositions 5 and 7)
- If you're inclined to build a more modest priced monument, consider building a sizeable pyramid, excavate a gigantic rock, or stack up old boats or cars and weld them together.

Build it, and your family and others will come…. far into the future.

41 PLANT A SEED

Consider becoming a Johnny or Josie Appleseed by planting trees, plants, and bushes in parks, forests or in any open space, public or private. Next to each plant, mount a small titanium or cooper plaque, dedicating it to yourself or someone living or deceased. Memorial spears can also be planted with the flora.

Trees should be given first preference, since they can live and give beauty for many centuries. Be *absolutely certain*, your plantings don't destroy or interfere with the surrounding vegetation.

- In your will or trust, note the location of plants.
- Start a family tradition of beautifying the world.
- As an alternative, create a small forest or orchard, where the public will be permitted to plant and dedicate a tree.
- Generally the public cannot plant trees on government land. Often permission may be secured in local parks.
- If permission is denied or you don't ask, risk planting in remote but accessible river, canal or lake banks and mountain and desert tracts. If you're queasy about placing a plaque, bury a spear. Be sure to plant away from areas of great public use. You could risk being fined, so be careful.

See Appendix to find out about memorial spears.
Read Proposition 29.

42 SHELTER ANIMALS

Consider building permanent or temporary shelters for domestic and/or wild animals. Each shelter should have your name, trademark or family coat of arms stamped on it. Shelters could be dedicated to different family members, friends, living or deceased.

Donate animal shelters to foster homes, Ronald McDonald houses, abused children's homes, boys and girls clubs, senior retirement homes or to any animal lover who wants an animal, but cannot afford to house it. Don't forget animals requiring hutches, aquariums, pens and cages.

- Build distinctive shelters for birds and small wild animals. Place them in the wild, where they won't interfere with the environment.
- In your will or trust, note the locations of your shelters.
- It's critically important to encourage your family and descendants to perpetuate a tradition of animal shelter charity. A monetary legacy might be an important incentive.

Do not shelter this idea from the public. Encourage participation!

> *"If we can devote ourselves to a cause or belief larger than ourselves, we can—in some small way—achieve a slice of immortality."*
> **Richard Leider and David Shapiro...20th century writers, career experts**

43 CARRY ON THE CAUSE

Consider placing in your will or trust, a challenge to heirs and descendants to continue your protest, fight or vigil. Set down your goals, and if possible, fund the effort to win your battle. With a sufficient legacy, heirs and descendants will have the means and hopefully the inspiration, to continue your vigil. If a monetary legacy isn't possible, hopefully your energetic drive in pursuing your cause will be a enough of an inducement for your descendants to continue your cause.

- The "fight" or protest might be for or against any public or private issue. It could range from a battle against an unjust employer to a world wide issue like nuclear disarmament.
- Many seek justice (a pardon) to exonerate themselves or a family member unjustly convicted of a crime. This process can take decades...even centuries. Even if the true culprit is found, pardons are extremely difficult to obtain.
- In your will or trust, specify the forum you wish to use—courtroom, media and/or public demonstration.

True story: My client was arrested for a crime committed by his brother. The client pled guilty to shield his brother from criminal prosecution. In his father's will, he granted a legacy to anyone who obtained a pardon for his son. After many years they succeeded.

Make your legacy...NEVER GIVE UP...

> *"I long to believe in immortality... If I am destined to be happy with you here—*
> *How short is the longest life? I wish to believe in immortality—*
> *I wish to live with you forever."*
> **John Keats, 19th century English poet**

44   LEGENDARY DEEDS

Consider creating a family legend by challenging heirs and descendants to accomplish a very specific physical or mental feat. If they do, they will be rewarded with a specific inheritance.

The physical accomplishment might be achieving All American status while playing varsity football for a specific college team, winning a named marathon, climbing a certain mountain or swimming a specific body of water.

The mental challenge to your descendants might comprise of achieving a PHD at M.I.T. *and* a law degree at Harvard. It is the stuff that makes legends.

- Provide a trust fund for those who accomplish the challenge. Be specific which bloodlines are eligible.
- By definition, legends should last forever. Make the Challenge, the stuff that makes people immortal.
- The challenge can require your heirs to do many deeds. You might require your heirs to graduate with a law decree from South Dakota University Law School...not Harvard. But they also must win the Boston Marathon.

Make your heirs and ancestors legends...as well as yourself!

45 FAMILY RITUAL

Consider establishing a family or personal ritual, which will be deeply engrained in family tradition and be continued by each generation.

Many family holiday celebrations and customs, both religious and secular, can become legendary, *if constantly repeated*. Family customs and rituals often change in time, becoming less strict in observation and often fade into obscurity. Only by strictly adhering to ritualistic procedures that you establish, will future generations continue the family tradition.

Some common traditions are to raise and lower the flag each day and decorating your home for the holidays. Establish a new one!

- Consider: observing a day of silence each week, a day of fasting each month, or doing a lawfully wild act once a year. An Ohio family catapults a junk car once a year.
- In your will, trust and/or autobiography, exhort future generations to continue the ritual. If able, give a legacy to family members who continue it.

True story: Some Hasidic Jews wore squirrel or other animal fur hats more than two hundred years ago. This tradition continues today.

Conduct religious holiday rituals…and your descendants will continue doing it.

> *"Higher than the question of our duration is the question of our deserving. Immortality will come to such as are fit for it and he would be a great soul in the future, must be a great soul now."*
> Ralph Waldo Emerson, 19th century American philosopher

46   PASS THE ZITHER

If you are an expert in a unique skill, craft or art form, consider passing your knowledge to the next generation. They in turn will pass it on and on...In your will or trust, reward those heirs and descendants who have mastered the skill or craft.

Contract with an established law firm, bank trust, C.P.A firm or other bonded agency to determine whether your heirs and descendants have mastered the craft. Give specific instructions on how to test the level of accomplishment.

- Do you have expertise in zither playing, archery, weaving, chess, cricket playing, organ grinding, bookbinding, bridge, vegetable art, orchid growing, wine making, Thai cooking or fly fishing? The list is endless. Pass the knowledge...
- As an added incentive for descendants to learn, pass the instrument of your passion (zither, chess set or fishing rod) to the heir who best master's the craft or skill. Be sure to engrave your name on the instrument.
- If your skill is professional, doctor, lawyer or dentist, be sure to pass the "tools of the trade" [scalpels, law books or drills] to the heir who achieves a mastery of the profession. Create a family legacy of masters.

Checkmate. BULLSEYE. Pass the knowledge on and on and on...

> *"From delusion, lead me to truth. From darkness, lead me to light. From death lead me to immortality."*
> The Upanishads, a treatise, part of the Hindu liturgy, written by Sanskrit, 800 BC

47 COAT OF ARMS

Consider creating a family flag or coat of arms if one doesn't exit. Focus on family history and traditions. If family members have a history of practicing a certain profession or if they're experts in a sport, craft, or trade, a coat of arms or flag should reflect these accomplishments.

Coat of arms and flag replicas could decorate your home and be sewed on family clothing. Smaller versions could be inserted into memorial spears or memorial canisters.

- If properly preserved, flags or a coat of arms can last for centuries.
- In your will or trust, reward descendants who fly the family flag or wear the coat of arms. Print the coat of arms on your will/trust.
- If you use your coat of arms in a business, be sure to apply for trademark protection with the United States Department of Patents and Trademarks.

Fly the legendary family flag ...wear the legendary family coat of arms, and other generations will follow. Need information on trademarks? See Appendix.

48 | COIN YOU, STAMP YOU

Consider designing and minting a coin or designing and printing a stamp made with the image of yourself or someone living or deceased. Coins can be produced in vast quantities or singularly. If you aren't interested in coins, consider stamps. Stamps will be easier and less expensive to make and duplicate.

To preserve your coin or stamp, place them in airtight receptacles like canisters and burial spears. Bury them or place them in a pond, lake or ocean. Stamps must be printed on acid resistant paper. Coins must be made with alloys or metals that will not rust. Nickel is nice, silver is good, but gold is best.

- Give the coins and/or stamps to heirs, family members, descendants, and friends. In your will or trust, provide a list of those descendants/ bloodlines who should receive these gifts. In your will/trust, list the locations were coins and stamps can be found or set up a treasure hunt.
- There are private mints and specialized printers that can do this work. Need help, See Appendix.

Coin one… stamp one…forever

49 AN IMMORTAL CAST

Have an outstanding physical feature—nose, ears, chin, biceps, hands, feet or privates? Consider casting it for posterity. Write on the cast your name and the date. The cast must be preserved and maintained so it will last hopefully forever. Do members of your family have any remarkable features? Cast them.

Generation after generation will have a unique view of your proboscis, hands, feet, ears or other large, small or irregularly shaped appendage. They will be able to compare the changes in body parts...evolution at work! Since you are the first to cast an appendage, your legend is assured.

- Family portraits and photographs should be included with the casts. Although these will give future descendants an image of you, having a cast, will be far more poignant.
- In your will/trust, give bequests to heirs and descendants who preserved yours and your family's casts. Also gifts might be given to those who add to the family cast archive. Don't forget to cast or get prints of your baby's or child's feet or hands. This is far better than bronze baby shoes.

Do you wear a size 9 hat or a size 18 E shoe? Those sizes may be small in 2050.

> *"For the last twenty five years, every Friday at five o'clock, I come here to drink three Budweisers and two hot dogs, with onions and mustard, while sitting on this bar stool. Its made me immortal around here."*
> Hannibal Z. Crawford, a 20th century beer lover, at a local bar in Fort Lauderdale, Florida.

50 A FOND FAREWELL

Consider throwing a final farewell party to celebrate your life or the life of your parent, child, sibling, relative or friend. A fond farewell party is appropriate only when the honoree has a limited time left to live.

Do not let illness, infirmity or vanity be an obstacle. This affair is not meant to be morbid or a search for sympathy. It should be a joyous celebration of the sweetness of life.

At the party, play desired music, serve favorite foods and give memorable gifts to friends and family. Plan a farewell speech, announcing what plans you are doing to become immortal. It's an important event so video it, so it can be distributed to future generations.

- A family tradition will be established, by granting a legacy to heirs and descendants, if they give a comparable farewell party. A hundred years from now, your great, great, great, great granddaughter may be saying her fond farewell, because of what you started.

Adios, bon voyage, ciao...

FINAL NOTES ON BEING IMMORTAL IN THE FAMILY

Most people will leave their estate to their immediate family. Their heirs will divvy up the "booty", shed tears for the departed and in a wisp of time, their memory will have vanished forever. You have an opportunity for your family to continue your flame forever. Use even a small part of your estate, to insure some measure of immortality for yourself, your family or a person living or departed. The main objective of these Propositions is to create legends, traditions, and myths. At the very least it could perpetuate your name or your essence forever. When legends are created, names will be remembered far, far in the future.

If you want to give all your money to your family without conditions and challenges…don't fret. You still can be immortal by doing some of the following: (a) execute and file an immortal will with a complete family history in Probate Court, (b) create treasure hunts, (c) bury memorial spears or memorial canisters (d) plant many trees with name plaques, (e) cast an appendage, (f) paint a self portrait or write an autobiography or biography of someone living or deceased or (g) execute any of the many Propositions we have set out for your consideration which require minimal expenditures. Choose to become an immortal. It will be the most important gift you'll ever give to your family.

May your family speak your hallowed name forever.

53

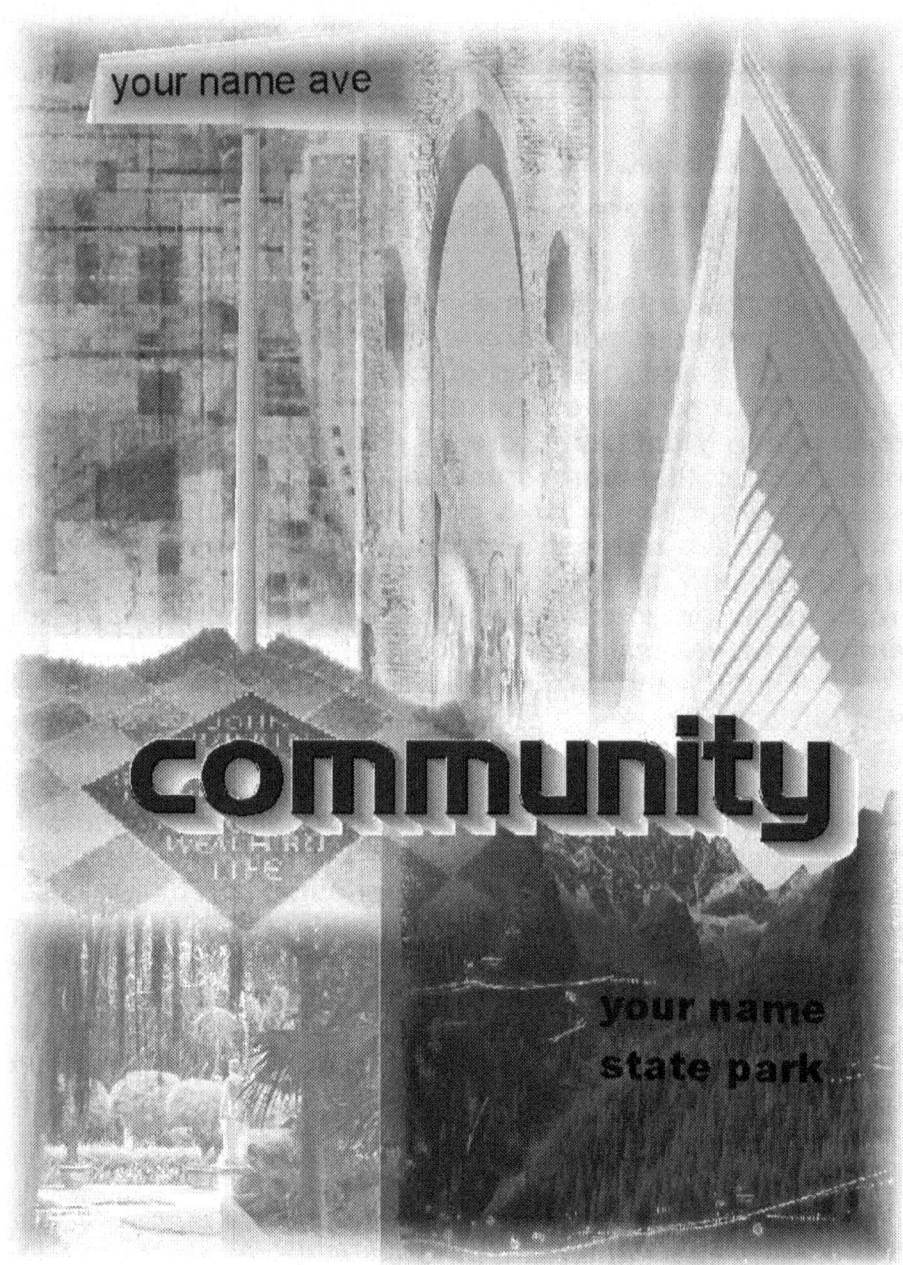

your name ave

community

your name
state park

PART II

ACHIEVING IMMORTALITY
IN YOUR
CITY OR COUNTY OR STATE

In Part I, you were asked to *consider and execute* various Propositions to achieve immortality within the family. In Part II, the focus is on expanding your immortal goals, by being remembered by the citizenry in your town, city and/or state. In executing these Propositions, please consider the following recommendations.

Many of these Propositions have a charitable quality. You can use your will and trust as legal vehicles in executing these Propositions. Consider a charitable trust, a non-profit corporation or a foundation. Seek legal advice to determine which legal medium is best suited for your individual situation. Careful planning is essential.

Secondly, I unconditionally recommend you attach your name, your family's name or the name of a loved one living or deceased to your charitable project. Many people sponsor charitable enterprises *anonymously.* I believe anonymous giving is a futile exercise in humility, a selfish need for privacy and most important, has no immortal impact. When a name is attached to a charitable endeavor, people identify that name with the charity. I *can think of no useful purpose for anonymous giving.*

There are several factors to consider when choosing any of these propositions. It is easier to achieve many of them within smaller communities. There will be less "red tape" to deal with. Yet, be mindful, cities might have a greater variety of immortal opportunities. Money will be an issue in many cases. Be realistic. Creative talent is important. Tenacity is absolutely essential. Can you ever become immortal? Yes, please try.

51 BUILDING FOR IMMORTALITY

If you are enamored with steel and concrete, consider having a building constructed or buying an existing building. Designate how the building is to be used. It might be for public use. That would be very special. Be *certain your name or family's name is etched on the edifice.* The building does not have to be a marble, pillared structure. A modest, but very solidly built park shelter will do. Imagine having your name on a structure for centuries.

- In time, the building may be designated as being historic and be preserved by the government forever.
- If the building is to be constructed after your death, in your will or trust give specific instructions as to how the building should be built and how it is to be used. To your will, attach architectural plans.
- If you are constructing a building for commercial use, it's likely your heirs will eventually sell it. The new owners will want to change its name. You may wish to give heirs the property on condition the name on the building remains the same. Also place the name restriction in the deed. (See Proposition 7).

Remember there are structures that have lasted since the time of the Bible. Yours could last longer.

52

LIBRARY ROOM
QUIET PLEASE!

If reading is your passion, consider organizing and/or funding a project to construct and equip a "special room" at a small or medium sized library. The room should have books and materials centered on one subject: cooking, travel, law or gardening. The room must be *distinctive* from the library itself.

Name the library room for yourself or for someone living or deceased. Condition the room's construction on a written contract with library overseers; that the room's name will never be changed.

- If you want the library room to be interactive, arrange for experts to give seminars demonstrating their skills.
- If you have written an autobiography, condition your "room gift", on the library keeping copies of the book on its shelves.
- If you don't have funds for a room, but you do own an unique book collection, donate them to a college or any institution. Condition the gift on the books being housed in a room you can name.
- If you have a large and, varied collection of books, start your own library. It is best to execute this project in a small town.

Leave a permanent "bookmark" in your community.

> *"I am thinking of auras and angels, the secret of durable pigment, prophetic sonnets the refuge of art. And this is the only immortality you and I may share my Lolita."*
> Valdmir Nobolov, 20th century Russian novelist

53 MUSEUM BOUND

Whether you collect antique toys, medieval armor or have an extra Rembrandt hanging in the attic, consider donating your treasure(s) to a museum. Condition your offer with name recognition on the exhibit, preferably, a biographical bronze placard.

When museum shopping, find a museum willing to give you the maximum immortal impact. Simply stated: what will the museum do to enhance your immortality? A special exhibition might be nice!

- Insist on a written pledge from the museum, that your donated piece will remain in their permanent collection forever and be exhibited continuously.
- Do you want to donate your treasure after death? Then in your will or trust, set out detailed instructions on how the gift should be donated, and which museum should receive it.
- You may be tempted to sell your piece to a museum. Be sure the "deal" doesn't compromise your immortal goals. Take a little less, to achieve more of your immortality objectives. Your name will last far longer on this planet, than the money you and eventually, your heirs will receive.

Have a rare antique? Allow endless generations to enjoy it.

> *"If we were to destroy in mankind the belief in immortality, not only love but every living force maintaining the life of the world would at once be dried up."* Fedor Dostoevsky, 19th century Russian novelist

54 | UNIQUELY SCHOLARLY

Consider establishing a college, graduate school or trade school scholarship for "special students." Rigidly restrict eligibility for the scholarship, to students who meet your eligibility requirements. This arrangement will keep the scholarship endowed for endless semesters.

Please note, donating large sums of money earmarked for a general scholarship fund may be laudable, but it is strongly discouraged. This charitable expression has no immortal impact.

- Set up a scholarship strictly for students born in a certain city neighborhood, or a town with a small population. Or limit eligibility to those students with unusual physical traits: red hair, six fingers, very small bodies or very large ones. There are plenty of scholarships available for those with big brains.
- How about giving scholarships to the magically inclined or clairvoyants? They might be highly successful in medical school and/or law school.
- Often parents establish scholarships to honor a child who died tragically. Establish the scholarship focused on what the child did or loved in their lives. Make it unique.

Establish a piano scholarship, for six fingered people and be remembered.

55 RESEARCH MYSTERY

Consider providing funding for a research project on a subject of great mystery and limited empirical knowledge. Gear your project to solving unknowns that will take researchers countless years to solve...but when solved, the resolution might have substantial immortal impact.

With intriguing subjects, and a *significant donation*, you likely will be able to affiliate with an established college, medically related facility or civic or religious institution.

- Consider: extensive research on haunted houses, war battles not mentioned in history books, proof of alien visitation, discovery of extinct cities or tribes, time travel, cures for extremely rare diseases, positive proof of afterlife, and the existence of mythical creatures bounding around the Earth, leaving large foot prints. Let your imagination abound, when designing your research project. Only then, will it last.

Like to find proof there are aliens among us? Be careful what you wish for.

56 HONOR THE LOST

Consider sponsoring a local special day to honor those who died in a specific natural or criminal event and *whose bodies were never recovered.* Honor those who died from a *specific* avalanche, hurricane, tornado, flood, tidal wave, earthquake, blizzard, terrorist attack, airplane sabotage or any calamity caused by a criminal act. Teaching the public how to survive a similar event, could be part of the program. Choose the day!

- If possible, a monument should be erected in the area the calamity occurred. The monument should be engraved with the names of those who were lost. Your name or the name of the person lost, should be prominently displayed.
- Establish a charitable trust or non-profit corporation to run this special day and raise funds to perpetuate it. To achieve your immortal objective, instruct your heirs and descendants to continue this sacred tradition. In this way, your name will always be linked to the day of remembrance.

Memorialize the lost and generations of their families will remember you.

> *"Beauty is momentary in the mind the fitful tracing of a mortal But in the flesh it is immortal, the beauty dies, the body's beauty lives."* Wallace Stevens, 20th century American poet.

57 | SINGULAR COMPETITION

Consider sponsoring a perpetual competition. It must be *distinctive* in scope, well funded, and attract a wide spectrum of contestants. Provide an exceedingly attractive prize. Decide how often it will be held, the criteria to determine a winner, the entity that will run the contest and the prize.

Many contests focus on writing, musical skills or testing physical or mental prowess. Unless these familiar contests have a solid financial base and are firmly established in the community, they may be doomed from the start. To achieve perpetual playoffs, the competition must be unlike any other.

- How about "Solve A Crime Competition?" The competition would be geared to solving serious crimes, the police have failed to unravel. When the crime is solved, a prize is earned.
- Or..."Solve the Problem Competition." Choose a problem adversely affecting the entire population of a town, city or state, that's unsolvable...Solve it and everyone wins.

Amateur sleuths...get on the start line and rive up your magnifying glasses.

> *"I don't want to achieve immortality through my work.*
> *I want to achieve immortality through not dying."*
> Woody Allen, 20th century American humorist, director

58 DEBATE IT

Consider initiating a lecture and/or debate series centered on inimitable themes. Political, legal and medically related issues are always of interest to some. Do not forget less debated topics: the occult, modern myths, or time travel are seldom debated and will always attract an audience. There is a plethora of talkers on the latter subjects but scarcely any forums.

Decide the perimeters of the lecture/debate series and how often it will be held. Name the series after yourself or any person you choose. [You can even designate whether refreshments will be served.]

- Offer a monetary grant to an educational institution, or an established civic or religious institution to *perpetually* sponsor the named debate/lecture series.
- To keep the lecture series perpetually alive, money is a truly tested fuel. Seek grants and tax deductible donations.

True story: A lecture series I was close to was the Frank J. Battisti Lecture Series at Case Western Reserve University. It was named for a Judge I clerked for. I don't think he was a fan of ghosts, goblins and time travel.

Talk, talk, talk, talk, talk...forever.

> *"The great ones, time never ends for them. Immortality is real when it comes to those people."*
> Al Davis, 20th and 21st century football coach and owner speaking of Sid Gilman

59   BE A SPORT

Consider creating a sports related charitable project. For maximum immortal impact, build a playing facility exclusively for a less popular sport. There are few public facilities in the United States for lacrosse, croquet, rugby, cricket, badminton, or lawn bowling. Are you interested in creating a community fishing pond or a cheerleading field? These projects may generate extraordinary community interest.

After your facility is completed and *named,* find an entity such as a city, a church, a civic group to perpetually maintain it. Don't be surprised if they want naming rights. But keep your immortal objectives on tract...DON'T GIVE IT TO THEM.

- You may attain immortality by building a popular sport community facility for baseball, football, tennis, basketball or golf (how about a free driving range or a par three golf course.) If the facility is well endowed, and your name is attached, your goal to be immortal, likely will be achieved.

Tennis anyone? The community will "love" it...

> *"Our creator would never have made such lovely days and given us the deep hearts to enjoy them, unless we were meant to be immortal."*
> Nathaniel Hawthorne, 18th century American novelist

60 IMMORTAL PARK

Consider creating a public park. Acquiring land is obviously essential, though many parks require only a large building lot. The most daunting task is to attain necessary approval from the government. Environmental and zoning are difficult issues.

Smaller tracts are ideal for parks geared to playing chess, picnicking, and for children's play- grounds. An urban park offering the public first-come-first-serve a variety of gardening opportunities, will attract many gardeners with hoes-in-hand. Larger tracts can be utilized for a variety of recreational uses from hiking to horsing around. There are many nude beaches, but why so few nude forests? Establish one!

- Lobby to secure perpetual government support for your park so they'll be responsible for perpetual maintenance. If a governmental entity won't accept your park, try linking up with a religious, civic, or a private corporation. Be sure to reserve the naming rights!

If you're creating a hiking park for nudists only, keep thorn bushes away from the trails.

61   ANIMAL ACTS

Consider creating an animal related charity that is accessible to the public. Government supported zoos, will gladly accept the public's donations and allocate those funds to their general fund. In this realm, the best immortal opportunities require a substantial gift for a single project. Below, are animal-related projects, with modest investment.

- Provide land for a free pet cemetery. It can be offered to the public with volunteer supervision or as a local government entity. If the government wants it, be certain your naming rights are preserved.
- Buy and maintain an unusual breed of animal. Be sure to allow public access for viewing.
- If there is no humane society in your town, establish one.
- If there is one, offer to fund a needed building addition. Condition your gift, by having naming rights to the structure.
- Obtain a very rare animal, and offer it to a public zoo.
- Some zoos allow donors to have their name etched onto a brick on a walkway. These projects raise substantial sums but have minimal immortal impact. Still, be sure the zoo will maintain the bricks. There are brick streets in many cities that have lasted centuries. Even a small immortal opportunity should be explored.

Own a white gorilla (better make that two) and make them and you immortal.

> *"All men's souls are immortal, but the souls of the righteous are both immortal and divine."*
> Socrates, Greek philosopher

62 THEATER BUFF

Consider donating a building, home, barn and/or land for a local theater and/or film project. Embark on a program promoting it. Establish a non-profit corporation to seek a solid and hopefully perpetual funding base. This project offers many opportunities for donors to receive immortal considerations including the chance to have a film or theatrical project dedicated to them. If you desire your project to begin or be completed after your demise, specify your intentions in your will.

- Your community theater project might focus on one aspect of the theater: children's plays, musicals, dramas, comedies, or ethnic plays in foreign languages. Your theater's uniqueness is an immortal imperative.
- If don't have the funds or financial support to establish this kind of charity, be the founder of a theater group connected with an established religious or civic institution. For naming rights, offer your services.
- Since films can be preserved for potentially centuries, this is a medium with special immortal opportunities. Producing films such as a documentary can have historical importance.
- You may wish to limit the project to creating screenplays and theatrical plays only. (See Prop. 64)

To be or not to be an immortal, that is the question.

> *"It has been drummed into man that he's mortal, but faced with something that really threatens to take away his right to immortality, he will resist as if he were about to be killed."*
> Andrew Tarkovsky, 20th century Russian film maker

63 MUSICAL LEGACY

Consider being the originator of a distinctive music related project. You can start the project by renting a facility, but to establish a lasting legacy, purchasing a building and land may be necessary.

For immortal impact, limit the project to a unique musical *situation.* For example, hard rock or country bands playing classical music, jazz quartets featuring bagpipe soloists, barbershop quartets that mix gender, ethnic groups or physical diversity and dance ensembles who kick and strut with or without clothes.

- A non-profit corporation, charitable trust or foundation should be created to fund the music project. An affiliation with a college or music school might be desirable.
- To avoid owning or renting a building, seek a joint musical venture with a well-established civic or religious institution. Naming rights must be assured.
- If the project is entirely independent, require project participants to generate income for the project, by selling recordings, teaching or providing entertainment.
- A recording studio or a composition component would be a splendid addition to the project.

DO RE MI…forever.

> *"The thought of being nothing after death is a burden insupportable to a virtuous man; we naturally aim at happiness and cannot bear to have it confined to our present being."*
> John Dryden, 17th century English poet

64   WRITING HOUSE

Consider being the founder of a Writing House. Support writers while they develop their craft or until they finish their writing projects. You can restrict the House to poets, novelists, or any literary specialists. If public funding isn't involved, access can be limited to writers of specific races, genders, sexual orientation, ages, religions, or nationalities.

- There are many Writing Houses throughout the country. If this Proposition appeals to you, visit several Houses and incorporate the ideas with your distinctive viewpoint.
- You can establish a Writing House by deeding your home, condominium, or commercial building to your Writing House non-profit corporation. You may be required to have a zoning and/or licensing commission approve your project. If you're deeding a condominium, the Board of Directors will have to approve the Writing House. These daunting aspects will be quite challenging. Advice from an attorney or city planner is recommended.
- To establish a Writing House posthumously, establish a bequest in your will or trust for that purpose. You may wish to give heirs a life estate in the property, and then the Writing House would follow their residence. See Proposition 5.

Discover a Hemmingway at home.

65 | AGELESS ART COLONY

Consider initiating an art colony dedicated to the creation of immortal art. Limit it to those artists who specialize in a specific medium or permit artists who dabble in various art forms. Painting and sculpture are the cornerstone art forms for most immortal art. You might consider gearing your project to the craft arts such as pottery making, crop art or woodwork. Also consider the designing arts like fashion, furniture making, jewelry design and architecture. Be sure to visit other art colonies with an eye towards your immortal vision.

- The creation of an art colony should begin with a building and be stocked with a full array of art supplies. Initial funding can be funneled through your non-profit corporation, charitable trust or foundation. It can be sustained by donations and by participating artists donating their work to the project.
- Set the rules governing your art colony, specifically entrance requirements, length of stay, and if any payment will be required by artists for their room and board.
- Require your portrait be prominently displayed at your art colony facility.

Does crop art and pottery making mix well for an artistic stew?

> *"The ultimate aim is to attain not only a state of healing, but eventually to bring ourselves to a state of incredible longevity. We might even reach the point of defeating death itself."*
> Herb Bowie, 20th century American writer

66 HUSH-HUSH CLUB

Consider being the instigator of a secret organization dedicated to creating legends...preferably your legend. Your secret society should have an altruistic element. For example, helping the poor fix their homes or cars *without being asked.*

Besides charity work and social activities, the secret society envisioned here, *must* have an active prankster component, for immortality purposes. Playing cunning, naughty, practical jokes on *public persons* can escalate the club and its most courageous members, into folk heroes. Over time, if the club's high jinks perpetrators allude being captured...Well, it's the stuff that creates legends.

- You being the founder of the secret society, will be assured your legacy, only if club members continue to talk, plot and act far into the night...having great fun.
- Your secret society should record their exploits for future generations to read and emulate.

Shhhhhh! The meeting of the secret order of the Blue Midnight Marauders is in session. Let the fireworks begin.

> *"Blow out your bugles over the rich Dead! There's none of these so lonely and poor of old. Sweet wine of youth gave up the years to be of work and joy and that unhoped serene. That men call age, and those that would have been their sons, they gave their immortality."*
> Rubert Brooke, 20th century American poet

67 INVENT IT

Consider endowing an Inventor's House. Provide amateur inventors with the opportunity to design a more diabolical mousetrap, a spectacular new pancake flipper or a _____!

Invention projects can be broad or geared to your specific area of interest. From airplanes to zodiac wheels, there is a world of want-to-be "Edisons" tinkering into the night. Providing a facility stocked with superior equipment is essential.

Set concise entrance criteria and rules for participation. Be sure the project shares patent and licensing rights. This will keep the project on an immortal course.

- Many inventors have created break-through inventions, but their names are often lost in obscurity. Why? Unlike Edison, they failed to attach their name to the invention. Be certain to secure naming rights for your inventors and yourself.
- By sponsoring an Inventor's House, you can become immortal without inventing anything.

There's a Hall of Fame for Inventors in Akron, Ohio. Perhaps, your Inventor's House will some day be prominently displayed.

68 | HALL OF FAME-GROUPS

Consider being the founder of a hall of fame for a local, well established religious, civic, educational, social or political institution or club. The project could be affiliated with a local or state chapter of a Lions, Elks, Veterans, or Kiwanis. If your community has no local sports hall of fame...establish it!

A community wide hall of fame honoring community activists of specific genders, religions, ages, ethnic backgrounds, or sexual orientation, could garner you considerable immortal impact. It will also give a measure of immorality to others.

- If the hall of fame you envision, was not started or not completed at the time of your death, in your will or trust provide funds to establish one. It may only require renovating a room in an existing building. Remember: set the guidelines how honorees gain entrance.
- Be sure honorees have more than a plaque. A photo and brief biography is essential. A marble bust or portrait with a biography is best.

Be sure your marble bust is featured.

69 HALL OF FAME-BUSINESS

Consider creating a hall of fame to honor people who are members of a specific profession, trade or job. Whether you are a business owner or a director of a profit or non-profit corporation, establish a hall of fame for employees. If there is no local or state hall of fame, honoring members of professions like medicine, law, accounting, teaching...start one!

Many organizations recognize employees with only pay increases and token promotions. A meaningful and permanent hall of fame would be a wonderful incentive to promote worker morale.

- Unions, trade groups, civic groups, political associations can honor members who helped build the group or association
- Professional associations (lawyers, architects, doctors e.g.) and various business associations are organized state wide, but few have established hall of fames. Urge them to do it!
- At the hall of fame site, provide sufficient room for busts or photographs and biographical plaques.

Did you know there is a Stripper's Hall Of Fame in the Mohave Desert? That institution gets to the bare bones of immortality.

70 UPSCALE SHELTER

Establish an upscale homeless shelter with an ethnic, educational or job related entrance requirement. Avoid infringing or duplicating the many established community shelters, like shelters that protect abused women and children. By rigidly restricting your shelter's entrance requirements, it will be both distinctive and separate.

The upscale shelter envisioned here, would provide superior food and lodging, along with amenities such as quality dental care, clothing, grooming and/or any service to renew a person's dignity.

- You might limit access to vagabonds, former graduates of a particular school, those born in a specific town or city neighborhood, or who worked in a certain profession or trade. Since those seeking help will have similar backgrounds, they may be able to help each other.
- The project's uniqueness should attract donations. You may need that element, to assure the shelter continuing. Only, a well-established shelter will insure your immortality.

Want to shelter vagabond graduates from your alma mater? They are out there.

71 FEED A NEIGHBOR

Consider instituting a feeding program that differs drastically from the generic soup kitchen or food bank. Instead of dishing out bland, boot camp chow, treat the homeless or other "needy" people, to a fine meal with blue ribbon service. In addition, offer participants a set of dress clothes, a hair cut and a shower for this singular occasion.

In this endeavor, eliciting the participation of restaurants, hotels and catering facilities might present them with an extraordinary chance for excellent free publicity. It is likely many can be persuaded to join.

Besides the meal, an optional spiritual or motivational message might have a positive affect on some of the diners. If it doesn't, at least the program will give them a fine dinner and a memorable evening and give you, legendary status.

- For maximum immortal impact, this program should run the entire year, and not just on holidays.

A delicious immortal idea! Can one fine dining experience change a life? Wouldn't it be nice...

> *"It must be so – Plato thou reason'st well! Else whence this pleasing hope, this fond desire, This longing after immortality? Or whence this secret dread and inward horror of falling into naught?"* **Joseph Addison, 18th century English essayist**

72   THE WINNER IS ...

Consider creating a *free* local raffle or lottery limited to a selected number of participants. The game of chance envisioned here, would allow only permanent, legal residents of a specific town or city neighborhood the right to draw a ticket. You can further restrict players, to those who belong to a specific civic, social, educational or religious group.

To be certain the raffle/lottery continues after your demise, allocate a specific bequest in your will or trust for future prizes and costs. Set forth instructions, as to who is eligible and how often the drawing will be held.

- This is a free-to-participate raffle, so the winner is essentially being given a gift. No gambling laws are being violated.
- No matter how often the raffle is held, if the prize is grand enough, the event will be momentous.
- If an original participant dies, his or her children should inherit eligibility. This condition would perpetuate the legacy.
- Establish the raffle (in your name) and endow it. Hopefully your descendants will continue it...forever.

Let them, spin the wheel...pick the number... and you'll be remembered forever.

> *"You can believe in God without believing in immorality, but it is hard to see how you can believe in immortality and not believe in God."*
> **Ernest Dimnet, 20th century French cleric**

73 JUST A LITTLE BIT

Consider giving the populace an opportunity for a *bit* of immortality. The idea is to provide an opportunity for a large number of people, a chance to participate in an immortal project. You being the founder of such a project will create great immortal impact for yourself. Below are a few ideas. Feel free to use them.

- Build and *maintain* a solid, stone eternal wall and inscribe the names of all residents who live in a specific village or town. As new residents join the community, their names should be added. This concept is applicable to residents living in a specific city neighborhood. Be sure your name or a name you choose is prominently displayed over the wall.

- Be the founder of a project designed to make others in the community immortal. Through a non-profit corporation, purchase video equipment and loan it out to those who want to create family histories. Promote immortality by offering citizens free burial spears and time capsules and educational materials.

- Provide and maintain a huge book near a famous community landmark. Offer residents and tourists an opportunity to sign their names and write a brief message. Over the years, the book will become a historical document. Generation after generation can check the book to see if their ancestors signed it. Your name should be on the cover.

Create bits of immortality for others and create an immortal mosaic for yourself.

> *"I love thee with a love, I seemed to lose. With my lost saints – I love thee with the breath. Smiles, tears, of all my life! – And if God choose, I shall but love thee better after death."*
> Elizabeth Barrett Browning, 19th century English poet

74   A MEMORIAL PARK

Consider building a memorial park dedicated to giving the public an opportunity *to honor a* family member or friend who perished in *a specific way*. Parks can be dedicated to those who died in car or airplane accidents, drowned, who were victims of crime or perished by a rare disease.

Parks could be devoted to several causes and sectioned out per cause. In the park, deceased families and friends could construct small memorials honoring loved ones.

- Grieving family members may find it easier to deal with their grief, by meeting with others who lost loved ones in similar circumstances.
- If you decide to dedicate your memorial park to multiple causes, the park will require a substantial amount of land. You must secure the approval of zoning and other government authorities. It will be a daunting task.
- In your will or trust, provide a bequest for park upkeep. If the park is properly maintained, these memorials should fascinate future archeologists.

Your memorial park should receive many donations and much help. A memorial park will remember the fallen, in a special way.

75 NAME A STREET

Consider being the founder of a group or organization to lobby local government officials to pass a law, giving citizens naming rights to public buildings and property, *for a fee.* As part of the legislation, you should seek city or town councils to appoint a citizen's commission to determine the amount of the fee, based upon the importance of the property to be named. As part of this legislation, lawmakers should honor prominent citizens without a fee. This program would generate sufficient funds to support other worthy public immortality projects.

- Fire hydrants, manhole covers, curbs, park benches, sidewalks would generate a small fee. License bureaus, bike paths, tennis courts, individual courtrooms would be in the middle of the chart. Parks, courthouses, major streets, hospital wards, buildings, police or fire stations would be top shelf. Street names would remain the same, but an individual's name would be added to the sign in small print. [In some cities prominent citizens have streets named for them. In Hollywood, Florida, most Presidents have a street]
- If this program was successful, you should be rewarded with a prominent boulevard.

Want your name permanently affixed on a water tower? Start lobbying!

> *"Our dissatisfaction with any other solution is the blazing evidence of immortality."* **Ralph Waldo Emerson, 19th century American poet and philosopher**

76 | NAME A TOLL BOOTH

Consider being the organizer of a lobbying organization to lobby a state legislature to do what is proposed in Proposition 75.

The public would pay fees set by a commission to have their names or a name, they choose, emblazoned on the great multitude of nameless state properties. A No Fee Commission must be created to honor individuals with a named property, who provided great public service. The number of naming opportunities should generate vast revenues. This project might even reduce taxes.

- Nameless highways, buildings, turnpike rest stops, bridges, state police barracks and tracks of land bordering the turnpikes and roadways are ripe for dedication.
- Heroic veterans, long serving and/or vital government workers, outstanding citizens who might be forgotten *forever,* would be remembered *forever.*
- If this project is successful, the leader of this revered movement will indeed become immortal.
- If the state movement works...why not organize an effort to lobby the Feds! The Federal Government has *a few* buildings, and property (how about a nice tank) that needs naming.

Do you want your name on a turnpike tollbooth? It is possible.

> *"Oh, may I join the choir invisible of those immortal dead who live again."*
> George Eliot, 19th century English novelist

77 PASS A RESOLUTION

Consider forming a group or organization dedicated to lobbying your local or state legislative body to honor citizens with in-depth *legislative resolutions.* Each resolution must cite the person's accomplishments.

The majority of people honored with legislative resolutions are elected or appointed government officials, the politically connected or those who have achieved a modicum of fame. Thus many deserving citizens, who contributed much to their community, will be and have been forgotten. An active state or local non-profit organization lobbying for recognition of deserving citizens will insure for them and you a small measure of immortality.

- If you are the founder of a resolution organization, you may garner even greater immortality, than the people receiving a resolution.
- Copies of the resolution should be preserved on archival paper and given to descendants. A resolution kept in government records, will last longer, than any monument.

This project could be expanded into lobbying the United States Congress for Congressional resolutions. See Appendix for help for a final resolution.

78 NAME A MOUNTAIN

Consider creating a non-profit organization seeking naming rights of natural sites owned by private individuals, businesses, developers, government and non-profits.

There are a myriad of unnamed natural sites that could be named for individuals or families both living and deceased. Think of the endless number of lakes, mountains, ponds, caves, cliffs, woods, brooks, hiking trails, swamps, and sections of land along streets and highways that are not named.

The founder of this organization should rate naming rights to a mighty mountain and a long hiking trail.

- There are a multitude of natural sites and obstacles on a golf course that could be named...*including the holes themselves.*
- Use your non-profit corporation to solicit naming rights from private parties who own tracts of land. In exchange they would receive a tax-deductible donation. Corporations might give their naming rights to their man made lake or other natural properties in exchange for similar tax relief.

There are many "water holes" on a golf course. Many golfers might feel a bit of revenge, if their names were attached to these holes!

> *"The thought of eternity consoles for the shortness of life."*
> C.G. Malesherbes, 19th century French Statesman

79   A NEW CRUSADE

Consider starting an *entirely new* local or statewide non-profit corporation focused on promoting a singular crusade or charity. Many charitable causes began locally and evolved nationally like M.A.D.D (Mothers Against Drunk Drivers.)

By working and contributing to an existing charity or public crusade, you may reap some recognition, even a nice plaque. Generally, these kinds of accolades will be short in duration and minimally remembered...if at all.

By igniting your original "movement" and promoting it, you can attain the greatest immortal impact. Below, are crusading ideas. Feel free to use them.

- Begin a crusade to rejuvenate run-down sports facilities, polluted parks or fix up abandoned churches or temples.
- Is your community lacking cultural programs? Do some old cemeteries need cleaning up? Are there old monuments in need of repair? Raise the banner and start!
- *Start a crusade to bring the town meeting concept to your hometown or city. Use sports stadiums to allow people to speak and vote on various local issues.*
- If your crusade or new charity is successful, you are bound to receive proper recognition (at least a memorial).

Set one's imagination on crusade control.

80 A CHARITABLE APPENDAGE

Consider creating an adjunct project to a local or statewide well-established charity. The base charity must have secure funding, and a solid record of longevity. A written contract between you and the charity is crucial. The contract must set out that after your initial founding grant; the charity will perpetually fund and maintain the project. Naming rights must be guaranteed. Below are a few project ideas.

- Grant a bequest to a legal aid society. Separately fund lawyers who represent poor tenants and who work to improve housing conditions.
- Fund a Lighthouse For The Blind Project to provide Braille signs in public and private buildings, especially restrooms.
- Fund a program with public television. Allow five minutes for a daily poetry reading. You select the poetry.
- Provide funding for an essential piece of equipment for an existing hospital, humane society, or any public medical related clinic. To achieve maximum immortal impact, you must condition the gift, on the institution maintaining and replacing it, with your name plaque always attached.

Even a modest opportunity to be immortal is better than no chance.

> *"God created man to be immortal, The fame of the brave out lives him. His portion is immortality. What more flattering homage could we pay to the manes of John Paul Jones."*
> **Paul Henri Marion, 18th century clergyman officiating at J.P. Jones funeral**

81   SUE THEM

Consider filing and pursuing a lawsuit to a judicial decision, which will permanently impact, on state or local law or affect your community forever. The case might be a class action involving the tax structure or challenging a police action that evolves into an important civil rights issue. Many major cases began at the local and state level and became national in scope. Roe vs. Wade and Brown vs. Board of Education are examples of cases that are firmly deep-rooted in our law, and the *parties names* are firmly entrenched in our American history.

- Courts make law. If your case isn't a precedent when you are alive, it could become a precedent later.
- Law school students learn law, by discussing actual court decisions. Cases decided in English Courts in the 17th century and by American Courts in the 18th century are still studied. File your case, and it may be discussed forever.
- In your will, provide a bequest to fund ongoing litigation. Appeals can be argued for decades.

Lawyers can achieve immortality with one case. The Judge(s) who decide immortal cases will also attain immortal laurels.

82 IMMORTAL STOREHOUSE

Consider building a non-profit Community Immortality Storehouse. Offer the public the opportunity to store any or all of the following at no cost or a sliding cost scale: videos, photos, important papers, films, autobiographies, scrapbooks, family heirlooms, cassettes, c.d.'s, and genetic material: hair, blood, a tooth.

Set the rules, as to who can store items in your park and how much they can store. A computer is essential to keep track of the items in each person's storage unit.

- An immortality storehouse can be a resource center, where descendants can learn their family history.
- It's likely the immortality storehouse will be popular and expensive. You could seek to arrange joint sponsorship with local or state government, or a civic or religious institution to share maintenance costs. As a non-profit corporation, tax-deductible donations should be solicited.
- A distinctive (perhaps pyramid shaped) and solidly built building will give further credence to the immortality theme of the storehouse. However, if you have an old warehouse not being used...well, it's a beginning!

The founder of an immortality storehouse will undoubtedly become immortal providing it's firmly established in the community.

> *"I plan to live forever and one of these days I'll probably be wrong."*
> Douglas McArthur, American 20th century Army General

83   PASS A LAW

Consider creating a non-profit corporation, which actively promotes and aids the public in placing their proposed laws on the ballot by initiative petition.

Most village, city, county or state charters or constitutions grant to the public the right to place their laws on the ballot for a public vote. This right is conditioned on obtaining enough valid voter signatures on a petition. This difficult task is formidable and this project would aid that effort.

The project could be expanded to include recall petitions (removing public officials) and referendum petitions (voiding valid laws passed by the legislature).

There is potential for the leader of this kind of organization to achieve immortality. There are also immortal opportunities for the initiative petition leaders, if their names are attached to a law passed by the voters.

- In your will or trust, a specific bequest should be allotted to the project, so it will continue far into the future.

Want to pass a law? It wouldn't be easy, but immortality might be the prize.

FINAL THOUGHTS ON CREATING IMMORTALITY WITHIN YOUR COMMUNITY OR STATE

As you read through Part II, it is clear that sufficient financial resources are helpful in attaining your goal of immortality. The ability to raise money, energy, passion, and imagination are also important. Assuming you have some financial resources but don't have the time or energy to execute any of the Propositions, you can still be immortal. There are several avenues to consider, but only one do we endorse.

First, avoid contributing substantial amounts to a community charitable pool. In a community pool, philanthropists (both large and small contributors) band their funds together to donate sums to hospitals, arts, scholarships and other charitable enterprises. The community fund is the donor and not the individual. Your name is literally lost in the pool. These philanthropic entities may be vital to a community, but in these pages, only individual efforts at being immortal are applauded.

The easiest way to achieve immortality but unfortunately with low immortal impact is to go immortality shopping. Or in other words—spread your money around. Check out your immortal opportunities and spend money on various projects. This effort should earn you the most immortal impact for your dollars, with the least effort expended. Many of the plaques or metals you garner with your name or the names of others living and deceased will hopefully, be in existence for hundreds of years.

Again, for maximum immortal impact, I strongly recommend fully executing one of the Propositions in Part II. If you work hard enough, you don't have to have any initial wealth. You can raise the money. Being an initiator...is far better than being a contributor. Do this and your chances of being noted as a true immortal, as the poet says "will meet with unexpected success."

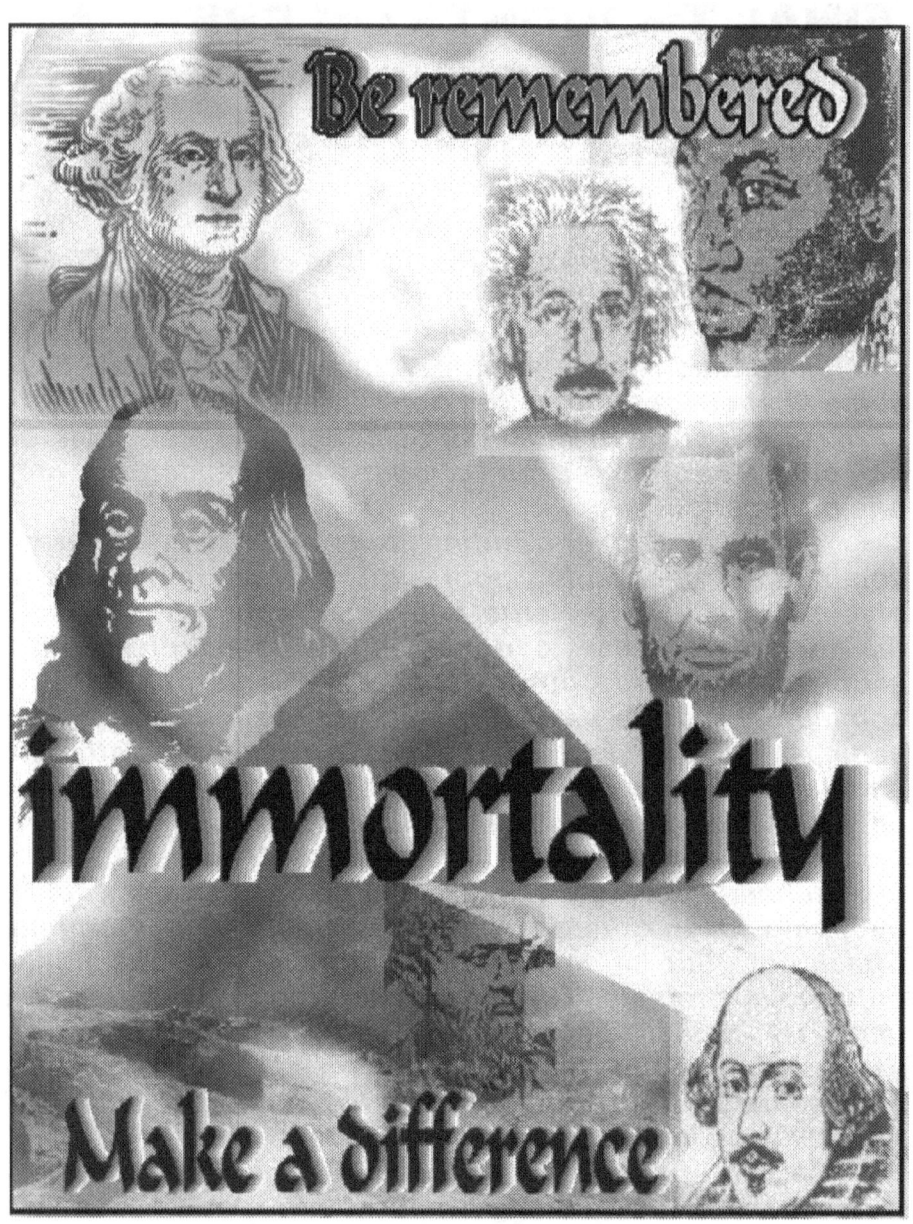

PART III

ACHIEVE YOUR IMMORTALITY NATIONALLY AND INTERNATIONALLY

In Part I and Part II, I encouraged you to fulfill as many Propositions as possible. I continue to do so. If you do, I am confident you will achieve some level of immortality. Throughout this book, I refer you to the Appendix in order for you to elicit our help in accomplishing your immortal goals. In Part III, the goal might be lofty but well worth the effort.

By completing just one Proposition, millions of people nationally and internationally may recognize your name for centuries. Let's be clear, very few will accomplish even a single Proposition...but you might.

Is it difficult to become immortal on such a grand scale? Absolutely! Is it impossible? Absolutely not!

We wish you the most profound luck.

Note: In this Part as well as the other Parts, the Propositions we've proposed are not conclusive. If you have an idea to become immortal, we'd love to hear it. If you need help to begin an immortal project, we encourage you to contact us.

> *"Our existence is but a brief crack of light between two eternities of darkness."*
> Vladmir Nabokov, 20th century Russian novelist

84   CREATE A FAD

Consider creating an innovative activity or product that evolves into a national fad. Generally, fads capture the public's attention only for a short time, but some do evolve and become a lasting part of our civilization. If your product or activity becomes global in scope, it may launch you into the immortal ranks. Below are a few *fad-making ideas. Use them!*

- Move the family or yourself to a ghost town or dense forest and write about your experience. Henry David Thoreau and other legendary characters did and their names will linger on forever. If your book causes a migration of people leaving the cities to experience a "freer life", this fad might be attributed to you. The result... your immorality.
- Create a national fad that results in people changing the way they conduct their lives. It can be a small thing. For example not using silverware. Eat caveman style in chic restaurants. Fly to work in a balloon. Hook up witnesses to lie detector machines, when they testify in court. That will cut down on litigation.
- Originate a word or phrase with your name attached to it. The word must be used in everyday language. The Earl of Sandwich's name has been around a few centuries.

Be careful flying a balloon to work in Manhattan.

85 | TRAGEDY MEMORIALS

Consider creating and planting a permanent memorial, a sculpture or a plaque honoring those citizens who were lost (died) due to a natural event. This memorial must be offered at least nationally but preferably worldwide. The natural event could have occurred any time in history. Your memorial should be planted even if a local one exists. Your memorial will be a permanent reminder of the tragedy for countless centuries. This Proposition should net you countless bonus air miles and immortality.

- Plant memorials where people died from an avalanche, hurricane, volcanic eruptions, tidal waves, floods, earthquakes, tornadoes, or forest fires.
- Memorials could be placed at sites of major airplane crashes, where ships were lost or at sites were people were lost in mountain expeditions or jungle explorations.
- In your will, encourage your descendants to continue your monument tradition. Provide financial incentives.
- This is a national or international effort, entirely separate from Proposition 56. This statute must be named for the founder (you). It would be like an Oscar of tragedy, but this profound memorial would honor the masses of the lost.

Become a student of history and plant your permanent Statute of Tragedy.

> *"Twenty three years old and I've done nothing for my immortality."*
> Fredrick Von Schiller, 19th century German dramatist

86 NEW NATIONAL CAUSE

Consider originating, advocating and leading an innovative national cause. Gun control, civil rights for various minorities, and a variety of environment movements can be traced from local advocacy that eventually became national and even international in scope.

In all countries, there are societal needs and injustices needing an infusion of leadership to correct. If one marches to the podium, others may follow. Below are a few of our ideas, as strange as they may seem. Yours may be better. Please see Proposition 79, which correlates well with this one.

- Advocate for a specific change in our United States Constitution and be successful in implementing it. For example, ban lifetime appointments for Federal Judges or create language that clears up the ambiguities in the Second and Ninth Amendments.
- Force manufacturers of noisy motorcycles, automobile boom boxes, leaf blowers, and loud car muffler to quiet their products or seek to nationally ban them.
- Require everyone to register their DNA...hair, a tooth, some skin, so people can be identified.

Dream up an idea, and get busy. Dreams take time to become reality.

87 | NEW POLITICAL PARTY

Consider organizing and leading a new national political party. Few have won an election for a significant public office running as a minor party candidate. Within the last decade, a Vermont Congressman and the Governor of Minnesota proved it could be done. Throughout history, a number of people have formed and led new political parties. The State's Rights Party, Socialist Party, Prohibition Party were just a few. Third Party leaders such as Henry Wallace, Norman Thomas and George Wallace influenced national elections and won something far greater...they're names will be in history books forever.

- Political parties have evolved over time, and many prominent ones, like the Whig Party in the early 19th century, are obsolete. So consider using an obsolete Party's name to advocate your issue. Reviving the name could attract your platform to media attention and leap you and your Party into the immortal ranks.
- By attracting media attention, your Party might attract money. Enough money and media, the big two in combination, and there's a slim chance to achieve this Proposition.

Bring back the Whigs! HAIR FOR ALL!

88   NAME ON A MAP

Consider buying a small town or village and name it after yourself, your family or anyone living or deceased. In the United States and other countries, there are many towns with zero or minimal populations. Many of these places are no longer on current maps. Review old maps and check government archives. You can find these towns and purchase them.

After buying or revitalizing a town, appoint yourself Mayor and sole law maker. Proclaim a law re-naming the town. In many jurisdictions, there is a process to have your town placed on a map. Put your kingdom on the map, and you'll likely become immortal.

- Another way to execute this Proposition is to buy land and develop a small municipality. This will obviously require a great deal of money. Buying even a dilapidated town may not be cheap. If you can't afford to buy a village in this country, try another country. There are lots of bargains in the jungle.
- Move your manufacturing plant to a small town with a weak economy. Condition the move, on the town being re-named with your name. Within the town's borders, there may be a mountain or lake with additional naming opportunities.

This Proposition may seem far fetched. It is not. I have a client who bought a small town in Texas with a very small population. He's re-naming it.

89 IMMORTAL INVENTIONS AND DISCOVERIES

Consider inventing, discovering or creating "something" that will improve the life of humans and/or animals. For maximum immortal impact, your discovery should be patented or the discovery fully documented. *The name of your creation must be identified with you.* Although your invention may be improved in time, or the discovery may lead to similar discoveries, the first creator or finder usually wins the ultimate prize... immortality. Below are a few invention/discovery suggestions.

- Devise a new game of cards, game of chance, or a sport with a different kind of ball. Create a sex-enhancing robot or any contraption that people will find enjoyment in using...for centuries.
- Create and name a revolutionary toy, food item, garment, musical instrument and yes a better mouse trap.
- Discover a new plant, lost civilization, new animal species, a new galaxy, or any creature or alien and name it.

Invent a new game using a triangle ball! Maybe someday a team from Mars will challenge Earthlings in the Galaxy Ball.

90 A NEW HOLIDAY

Consider creating a new holiday. Its origin can be secular or religious.

Mother's Day, Halloween, Valentine's Day, Father's Day and Groundhog's Day were all holidays, literally "dreamed up." The names of the founders of some of these holidays are etched forever in history. The challenge is to devise a new holiday, with a compelling reason to celebrate it. Below are a few frolicking suggestions.

- "GET HIGH ON LIFE DAY". No one works. Anyone can do anything outrageous, as long as it's legal... Raccoon Day instead of Groundhog Day, Abhorrence Day instead of Valentine's Day (send a "loved one" a batch of poison ivy) or more realistic possibilities...National Step-Parent or Foster Parent Day.
- Promote a holiday to honor a momentous event that happened in the past: Ten Commandments Day, Printing Press Day (celebrating the first printing press), Miracle Drug Day, (celebrating the discovery of life saving vaccines.) Dream up a day, and many may celebrate it...especially, if the populace receives a paid day off.

Get High on Life Day sounds uplifting.

> *"Despair and suicide are the result of certain fatal situations for those who have no faith in immortality its joys and sorrows."*
> Gerald de Nerval, 18th century French writer

91   OWN A COUNTRY

Consider buying or squatting on a small, unpopulated island off the United States shoreline or any similar island off the shorelines of many countries in the world. The island-buying and squatting possibilities are plentiful. Find one, buy or squat on it, name it and plant the family flag or coat of arms deep into your soil.

Seek recognition by any country near it, though this will be a difficult task to attain. By having your named island on some map, (even a nautical map), you will surely be marked... an immortal.

- Try exploring the buying possibilities of the many islands off the coast of the United States, Canada, Greenland, Africa, South America or Australia. In the Pacific Ocean, there are a plethora of islands that can be squatted on or purchased for modest amounts.
- If you can buy an island posthumously, set out the details in your will or trust. Be sure to provide a specific bequest so your executor or trustee can buy and name your island.
- You might gain title by squatting on an island off the U.S.A coast.. Open notorious possession, over many years, is the standard to gain title in most states. If the island is close enough to a state, then state law would govern.

Do you want to squat on an island? Bring plenty of vitamins and sunscreen lotion. Note: Proposition 86 might be easier, but this one is more worldly.

92   BE A FIRST

Consider achieving a momentous feat or a single record of human achievement, that no person has ever accomplished. Only the most extraordinary acts and records will be remembered forever. *Local* community records whether exemplary, like the longest tenure in office for an elected official or frivolous, like the greatest oral projector of watermelon seeds, may achieve a degree of fame for the record setter. However, these records are not within the perimeters of this Proposition.

Only the most astounding worldwide feats will be remembered forever. Below are some firsts, which when accomplished might be dubbed astonishing records by future generations.

- Be the first person to: dole out a million dollar in one dollar bills to a million people, climb the highest mountain in a hundred countries, earn a hundred college decrees including a M.D. decree from accredited colleges, climb the highest mountain the world and dive to the lowest depth in the ocean, walk across the United States while passing through its most notorious city ghettos ...and survive.
- Be the first to walk across a certain desert, swim across a certain sea, skate across a certain continent and if nobody has done it...do it!

Dream it up, do it and be remembered.

93 Spread Your Art Worldwide

Consider creating art for a specific audience, and sending your pieces worldwide.

For example, send your work to hospitals, especially if your work gives patients tranquility. Send your art to churches and temples to promote spirituality. If there is a humorous touch to your creations, share it with those who live in dreary places and need cheering up. By exposing your art to a specific audience, someday, somewhere, you may be discovered, and be resolutely proclaimed *an immortal.*

- Hang your paintings of courage in towns that have suffered from a natural or man made calamity, plant your sculptures of peace in places where there is constant war, hammer your art into cliffs of desolate places where they might be treasured and preserved by villagers forever.
- Your art might not be appreciated in your native country, but in Mozambique, you could be another Picasso.
- In executing this Proposition, talent is important, but tenacity and planning are essential. Remember your exposing your art to the world...at your cost. Invest your time wisely when gallivanting around the world, and pick the right places.

When hammering paintings into cliffs...be careful.

> *"I believe in immortality of the soul, because I have within me, immortal longings."*
> Helen Keller, 20th century American author

94 | WRITE FOR POSTERITY

Consider creating an immortal piece of writing: novel, autobiography, biography, poem, short story, comic, essay, non-fiction piece, theatrical play, screenplay or even a letter, "Yes, Virginia there is a Santa Claus".

Your written masterwork can vault you into the immortal ring. Emma Lazarus wrote "Give me your poor, your huddled masses yearning to breathe free". Her words are etched into the Statute of Liberty. It is her only truly immortal work. It's enough.

- If you find it difficult to get published, then self-publish. Many famous authors have self-published. Poe, Thoreau, Whitman are a few, who've met with "uncommon success."
- If you have written a book and are frustrated with its limited readership, try this plan. Acquire a large quantity of quality hard backed used and new books. Offer your books to small and medium sized libraries worldwide, with one condition. Your book(s) must be added to each of the accepting library's permanent collections. Perhaps in the future, a major critic will pick up your book, read it and declare it a "magnum opus."
- Set aside funds in your will to be certain your book is published. If you have only book "in you" make it an autobiography...the best book for immortal impact.

Send a copy of the book with an ISBN number to the Library of Congress.... They will keep it forever.

> *"One of the strange things about living in this world is, that it is only now and then one is quite sure one is going to live forever and ever and ever."*
> **Francis Hodgkin Barnell, 20th century American writer**

95 | BUSINESS REVOLUTIONS

Consider creating an entirely new industry or revolutionizing an existing one, that will be remembered forever.

If you can merge a world- shattering marketing idea, an indelible advertising program and/or an innovative financing scheme with products that will be in demand forever, your immortality is assured. It wouldn't be easy.

- A few companies on track to be immortal are the Golden Arches of McDonald that revolutionized the restaurant industry, Nike and its trademark, Coca Cola which has its own museum, Hershey, the synonym for chocolate and a company who's family name is synonymous with beer and budding flowers. Will these companies be around in future centuries? In my opinion, it is very likely!
- Many service industries from weight-loss programs to tax services will be remembered with the founder's name. When you think of mail order catalogs, two searing names immediately "buck up". If your name is attached to a popular service company or product, it increases the chances of you achieving immortality.

Even if your business is not a financial success, if you've left products that have a forever shelf life, your immortality would seem assured.

96 | COLLECT ALL OR ONE

Consider amassing an immortal collection of first editions, baseball cards, stamps, coins, paintings, dolls, cars, antiques, or other valuables (even bottle caps). For a collection to be adeptly branded with the *immortal tag,* it must be considered by experts as being one of *the* finest in the world.

Not interested in collecting, but owning one worldwide coveted object? Although the object might be extremely expensive or rare, *expensive or rare* alone will not reach the standard to accomplish this Proposition. Only by owning the rarest of objects will you or your family achieve worldwide immortality.

- In Proposition 6, it was proposed for you to accumulate and pass your rare collection or valued family heirlooms from generation to generation. Please still consider doing that! But in this Proposition the challenge is far more distinctive and difficult. to accomplish.
- By allowing public access to your collection or object, your chance to generate significant worldwide immortality will greatly increase. However, you may decide to shuck the level of immortal impact by keeping the object or objects solely within your family. Is that so bad?

Own a Maltese Falcon and be remembered.

97

A SONG, A DANCE
A FILM, A PLAY

Consider creating an immortal work of music, a dance, a film, a play, a TV show. There are very few pieces of performing art which over a long period of time will be stamped, *immortal*. A few of our *modern* picks for immortality are: the twist, I Love Lucy, Godfather, South Pacific, Death of a Salesman, the Beatles Song, *"Yesterday"*, and Cinderella.

Today, with most popular music being recorded on discs and most films being recorded on DVD, if your work is not initially popular, it has been preserved and could become a worldwide craze in 2050.

- Musicians and songwriters who want to write an immortal tune, consider: a holiday song (White Christmas or Elvis' Blue Christmas) a patriotic piece (Star Spangled Banner), a children's song (Old McDonald), a drinking song (A Hundred Bottles of Beer on The Bar), a sports song (Take Me Out to the Ballgame). If you write a song in these categories, it could be popular for centuries. Current popular hits are measured in months.
- Festival and ethnic dances will always be a part of human civilization. Devise a new dance to honor your heritage.
- Great documentary films will always have historical value. So will the greatest musical or theatrical plays...only the greatest.

Drink to Me Only with Thine Eyes is a four hundred year old song, that's still popular.

98 | A NEW IDEOLOGY

Consider creating a new ideology, cult, religion, or philosophy that causes a mass following. Your "following" might begin, by the public reading your book. From this beginning, a mix of excellent public relations and charismatic leadership can generate a *new way, a* popular way for centuries.

It is likely your new ideology or religion will not achieve mass support during your lifetime. Throughout history, those who led great religious or philosophical movements, never saw the universal acceptance of their work: Abraham, Jesus, Buddha, Martin Luther King. Today, with the multitude of media sources, there are opportunities to reach great numbers of people. Only a vast acceptance of your new way of thinking or believing will create immortality for yourself.

- There have been many false messiahs and cults that enjoyed a brief following, only to vanish without a whisper. Only a religion or ideology with continual crowd appeal will last forever.
- Have an idea for world peace? A new deity? A new political philosophy? In your will or trust, state how your spiritual movement should continue. Consider a monetary legacy.

Making your philosophy others' philosophy will be philosophically rewarding.

99   ONE ACT

Consider planning and executing a single act, or series of acts so great or so historic, you will be anointed by historians with the status of *an immortal.*

To illustrate this Proposition, most great sports achievers are immortalized in Halls of Fame by their play over a lifetime. Yet some players have Hall of Fame recognition, for having executed a single immortal act (or singular series of acts). Don Larson's perfect game, Bobby Thompson's home run, Tom Dempsey's field goal, Franco Harris' catch. These names will be remembered.

- Paul Revere's horse ride, Edmund Hillary's mountain climb, Nathan Hale's final words before being hung, John Wilkes Booth's assassination of President Lincoln (he is infamous, a loathsome kind of immortality, given to a few heinous criminals), Betsy Ross' knitting job, Charles Lindberg's and Charles Byrd's successful airplane "rides", Amelia Earhart's unsuccessful air excursion, and Neil Armstrong's walk are only a few immortal acts. Their names will likely be remembered forever.
- Many singular acts cannot be planned. Some may require your ultimate courage to survive a situation. Immortality may not be your initial goal, but you might have an opportunity to reach this glorious plateau. The timid will not achieve this Proposition, so act.

Are you ready if destiny calls you? It may!

> *"I know we live after death and again and again, not in the memory of our children or as a mulch for trees and flowers, however poetic that may be, but looking passionately and egocentricity out of our eyes".* **Brenda Ueland, 20th century American poet**

100 IMMORTAL CAREER

Consider striving to become an immortal. There is no loftier goal, and it is achievable. Many strive for and will achieve wealth, notoriety, or a modicum of political power. Some may even gain momentary fame. Yet, few will be universally known as being an immortal. Most famous people will lose their notoriety in a decade. The goal of achieving immortal status may seem impossible? At this level, the formula for immortality is to continually build a career of unwavering excellence in a field. Who is an immortal is debatable. A few of our picks are below.

- Acting: John Wayne, Katherine Hepburn, Paul Newman
- Singers: Frank Sinatra, Elvis Presley, Barbara Streisand
- Politicians: Franklin Roosevelt, Ronald Regan, Golda Meier
- Business: William Gates, Ted Turner, Sam Harkins
- Television: Lucille Ball, Jackie Gleason, Norman Lear
- Scientists: Jacques Cousteau, Jonas Salk, Albert Einstein
- Military: Moshe Dione, Dwight Eisenhower, Winston Churchill
- Composers: Irving Berlin, The Beatles, Richard Rogers
- and then it could be_____ you!

Who are your picks? We'd like to know..

APPENDIX

You can achieve immortality without any aid or advice. There is nothing to buy, nothing to own. You can do it on your own. But I believe you will be able to achieve immortality far faster and your efforts may be far more effective by contacting our company IMMORTAL SOLUTIONS.COM or E-mail us at Immortsol@aol.com. We have products and services to help you and your family, have presence on earth forever.

1. We have legal documents you can use to execute the appropriate Propositions: Immortal wills, name change kits, ethical wills, letters from the grave, cloning codicils, life estate deeds, and a C.D. on how to execute them. These can be used in all jurisdictions
2. We have products like remembrance stones, burial spears of all sizes including the mini-spear to wear or carry, clone stone jewelry, a baby dome and a glass dome (Oculus) to enhance your spiritual inclinations.
3. We have services to aid you in executing each and every Proposition in Parts I and II. No exceptions. The services include: legal services to execute documents, free referrals like finding an author to write or help write your autobiography or a loved one's biography, helping execute your plans for a private cemetery, planning and executing a campaign for you to achieve immortality, setting up a charity and even finding a proper medium for you to contact those who have perished.
Test us.

4   If you want to be remembered, have lost a loved one and want that person to be remembered; if you want to honor your entire family or someone living; if you want future generations to continue traditions you've established forever...contact us.

Web site: immortalsolutions.com
E-mail: immortsol@aol.com

Write us for our free pamphlet.
Immortal Solutions
4491 S. State Rd. 7 #314
Davie, Florida 33314

Call us at (954) 321-6669 if you are interested in our services. Don't forget to check our website for the first clue to our absolutely free chance at finding our buried treasure. It may take more than one clue, but It is worth finding. See website for additional free clues.

THANKS FOR READING THIS BOOK.
NOW IT IS TIME TO ACT!

ABOUT THE AUTHOR

Lloyd B. Silverman is the President and founder of Immortal Solutions Enterprises. The company is dedicated to creating the opportunity of immortality. It aims to inspire all of us "to become *immortal*." This opportunity is available to people of all ages and of all incomes.

He is a graduate of Ohio University and American University's Washington College of Law. He is a member of the Florida Bar and has been practicing law for 36 years.

The following is a list of the author's accomplishments in the legal field: He is an inactive member of the Ohio Bar and was a member of the Missouri and the New York Bar Associations. He was formerly a law clerk to Federal Judge Frank J. Battisti (deceased), Assistant Law Director of the City of Cleveland, Executive Director and Public Defender of the Stark County Legal Aid and Public Defender (Canton, Ohio). He was Executive Director of the Western Missouri Legal Aid (Kansas City and West Missouri), Director of the Bronx, New York Legal Aid Services, Senior Citizen Project Director with the Broward County (Florida) Legal Aid. He was appointed by Governor Bob Graham to be an Ombudsman in Broward County, Florida. In addition, Mr. Silverman was a lecturer at Akron University Law School and John Marshall Law School in Cleveland, Ohio.

"In his spare time", Mr. Silverman has spent the last eight years working specifically in what he calls "the world of immortality". He now dedicates his future and your future to becoming immortal.